Reactive Hypoglycemia Quackery

Exposing Myths and Dangerous Treatments

Cheryl White MAT

Dr. Shane Wilson.

Dedication

To all my friends and family who supported me through the ups and downs of reactive hypoglycemia and encouraged me to seek answers – thank you from the bottom of my heart.

1 Introduction

In the face of chronic illness, the pursuit of relief can lead patients down many different paths. When a diagnosis like Reactive Hypoglycemia (RH) is given—especially when it involves frustrating symptoms such as sudden drops in blood sugar levels and the need for constant dietary vigilance—it is natural to seek out alternatives. As patients and their families navigate the often complex and uncertain terrain of this condition, the allure of non-traditional treatments or so-called "cures" can become overwhelming. The internet, rife with self-proclaimed health gurus and alternative medicine advocates, offers a wealth of unregulated advice, much of which promises to cure or manage conditions like Reactive Hypoglycemia. But amidst the noise, how can patients discern real hope from harmful quackery?

This book, *Reactive Hypoglycemia Quackery*, aims to arm patients, their families, and healthcare professionals with the tools to critically evaluate the misinformation that surrounds Reactive Hypoglycemia. While there are legitimate medical treatments and management strategies for RH, none of them are quick fixes, and certainly none involve miraculous "cures" without careful dietary management and lifestyle changes. Yet, many patients—facing the frustration of fluctuating blood sugar levels, unexplained symptoms, and the lack of comprehensive information—turn to unproven and often dangerous alternative treatments. This book will delve into these quack treatments, exposing their fraudulent claims and explaining why they cannot work. In this introduction, we will explore the appeal of alternative treatments, the science behind Reactive Hypoglycemia, and why critical thinking is vital for patients navigating a sea of misinformation.

The Rise of Quackery: Why Are Patients Drawn to It?

Before diving into specific quack treatments, it's essential to understand why they exist and why they continue to thrive despite overwhelming evidence against them. Quackery—fraudulent or ignorant medical practices—has a long history that predates modern medicine. Historically, before scientific advancements in healthcare, patients relied on folk remedies, superstitions, and charismatic healers who promised miracle cures for ailments that medicine had no answer for at the time.

Fast forward to the 21st century, where technology has rapidly advanced our understanding of conditions like Reactive Hypoglycemia. While this has led to more effective management strategies, the rapid spread of misinformation through the internet has also fueled the growth of modern-day quackery. With a quick online search, patients are exposed to countless websites, blogs, and YouTube videos offering "natural" or "holistic" cures for RH, many of which are nothing more than rebranded snake oil.

Patients may be drawn to these false promises for several reasons:

1. **Frustration with Symptom Management**: Managing Reactive Hypoglycemia often involves constant dietary planning and monitoring blood sugar levels. The idea of a simpler, non-invasive alternative can be enticing, especially when patients struggle with the rigidity of conventional advice.

2. **Desire for Control**: Chronic conditions like RH can make patients feel helpless, especially when episodes of low blood sugar seem unpredictable. Quack treatments often give patients the illusion of control—whether through supplements, lifestyle hacks, or drastic diets—allowing them to feel empowered in managing their condition, even

if the approach is entirely ineffective.

3. **Emotional Vulnerability**: Living with a condition like Reactive Hypoglycemia, which can cause symptoms like shakiness, sweating, dizziness, and confusion, can be emotionally exhausting. Desperation for relief, combined with the mental toll of chronic illness, makes patients more susceptible to quick fixes and miracle cures, even in the absence of credible evidence.

4. **Misinformation and Pseudoscience**: The internet is rife with pseudoscientific claims. Many people lack the training or resources to distinguish between credible medical advice and unsubstantiated health claims. Some quack treatments are even backed by professional-looking websites, testimonials, or celebrity endorsements, lending them an air of legitimacy.

What Is Reactive Hypoglycemia?

Reactive Hypoglycemia is a condition in which the body experiences low blood sugar (hypoglycemia) within a few hours after eating a meal, typically one high in carbohydrates. Unlike other forms of hypoglycemia related to diabetes or fasting, Reactive Hypoglycemia is linked to an abnormal insulin response following meals. Symptoms may include dizziness, weakness, sweating, irritability, and confusion, and can range from mild discomfort to more severe, dangerous drops in blood sugar.

The exact cause of Reactive Hypoglycemia is still not fully understood, but it may be related to an overproduction of insulin by the pancreas in response to carbohydrate intake. Other possible causes include certain metabolic disorders, prediabetes, or conditions that affect how the body handles glucose. Diagnosis typically involves monitoring blood sugar levels and evaluating symptoms after meals.

What Science Tells Us About RH Management

Managing Reactive Hypoglycemia involves careful planning, particularly regarding diet. The goal is to prevent large spikes and subsequent drops in blood sugar. Eating smaller, more frequent meals that are balanced in protein, fat, and low-glycemic index carbohydrates is essential. Additionally, regular physical activity and avoiding excessive sugar and refined carbohydrates can help stabilize blood sugar levels.

While these approaches are proven to help manage RH, no supplement, diet fad, or "miracle cure" can reverse the body's underlying insulin response issues. Despite this, countless alternative treatments are marketed to patients, often with the claim that they can regulate blood sugar or "cure" Reactive Hypoglycemia entirely.

Case Study: The Dangers of Unapproved Supplements

A striking example of the harm caused by quack remedies can be seen in the case of Enzymatic Therapy, Inc., a company involved in selling unapproved supplements and making fraudulent health claims. Over a six-year period, the company falsely promoted products claiming to cure a wide range of illnesses, including Reactive Hypoglycemia. The FDA's investigation into the company began after consumer complaints of adverse reactions, including a death from one of their unapproved supplements. Despite repeated warnings from the FDA, the company continued to market products that had no scientific backing and, in some cases, led to serious injuries and death.

One consumer, after taking a supplement purporting to aid hypoglycemia, became violently ill, while others suffered tissue damage and elevated thyroid levels. The company's disregard for safety and the FDA's repeated warnings exemplifies how dangerous unregulated supplements can be, particularly for conditions like RH. This case highlights the importance of relying on scientifically vetted treatments rather than risking one's health on unproven and potentially dangerous alternatives.

The FDA ultimately shut down the company, banning them from manufacturing or promoting their products, but only after significant harm had already occurred. This case serves as a powerful reminder of the risks associated with unapproved, unregulated supplements that make false claims about their efficacy in treating serious health conditions like Reactive Hypoglycemia.

The False Promises of Diet-Based Cures

One of the most pervasive forms of quackery in Reactive Hypoglycemia treatment is the idea that certain diets can cure or reverse the condition. Popular fads include ketogenic diets, juice cleanses, or restrictive eating patterns that promise to "reset" the body's blood sugar regulation system. These diets are often promoted by alternative health practitioners or influencers on platforms like YouTube and social media.

While maintaining a healthy, balanced diet is critical in managing Reactive Hypoglycemia, it's important to understand that extreme diets—especially those that restrict entire food groups—can do more harm than good. The idea that a specific diet alone can cure a complex metabolic condition like Reactive Hypoglycemia is misleading at best and dangerous at worst.

For instance, the Mayo Clinic and other reputable health organizations often recommend more sustainable and well-rounded approaches like the Mediterranean diet for managing overall health, including blood sugar levels. The Mediterranean diet emphasizes whole grains, lean proteins, healthy fats like olive oil, and plenty of vegetables. This balanced approach helps stabilize blood sugar and provides long-term health benefits without the risks of extreme restrictions.

On the other hand, a meat-centered, high-fat European diet, which may rely heavily on processed meats, saturated fats, and refined carbohydrates, could worsen Reactive Hypoglycemia by causing sharp spikes and crashes in blood sugar levels. Diets high in unhealthy fats and low in fiber can exacerbate insulin sensitivity issues, leading to more frequent and severe hypoglycemic episodes.

Therefore, while the Mediterranean diet is a sound

approach that aligns with managing blood sugar, extreme diets that cut out essential nutrients or focus too heavily on unhealthy components can disrupt the delicate balance needed to keep blood sugar levels stable in those with Reactive Hypoglycemia. Patients should avoid the false promises of fad diets and instead focus on scientifically backed, balanced eating plans like the Mediterranean diet, which are proven to promote overall metabolic health.

Detoxification and Supplement Scams

Another common theme in RH quackery is the concept of detoxification—ridding the body of "toxins" to improve blood sugar regulation. Various detox diets, cleanses, and supplements are marketed as ways to "balance" the body and prevent blood sugar drops. These treatments often involve fasting, consuming large amounts of fruit juices, or taking expensive supplements.

The idea of detoxifying the body has become increasingly popular in alternative medicine circles, but it is based on a misunderstanding of human physiology. The liver and kidneys already do an excellent job of removing waste from the body. No external detox program can regulate blood sugar or address the root cause of Reactive Hypoglycemia.

Supplements marketed to RH patients often claim to support glucose metabolism or stabilize blood sugar levels. While some supplements, like chromium or magnesium, may have minor roles in blood sugar regulation, they cannot replace the careful dietary management that is required for RH. Worse, some supplements can interfere with other medications or cause unintended side effects.

The Role of Pseudoscience in Online Communities

One of the most insidious aspects of modern quackery is the role of online communities in perpetuating misinformation. Websites, forums, and social media groups dedicated to alternative treatments for Reactive Hypoglycemia can create echo chambers where unproven or dangerous treatments are promoted without scrutiny. These communities often dismiss mainstream medicine and instead promote alternative "cures" that lack any scientific validation.

YouTube and other video platforms have become breeding grounds for misinformation, with countless videos touting miracle cures for RH. These videos often feature testimonials from patients who claim to have "cured" their condition through dietary changes, supplements, or alternative therapies. However, these testimonials are anecdotal and lack the scientific rigor necessary to support their claims.

The Importance of Critical Thinking and Medical Guidance

As patients and their families navigate the complexities of Reactive Hypoglycemia, it is critical to approach all treatments—especially those found online—with a healthy dose of skepticism. The best way to protect oneself from quack treatments is to rely on credible sources of information, such as peer-reviewed medical journals, reputable health organizations, and consultations with qualified healthcare professionals.

Patients should always be cautious of treatments that:

- Promise a "cure" or quick fix.
- Rely heavily on anecdotal evidence or testimonials.
- Suggest that mainstream medicine is hiding the truth.
- Involve expensive supplements, detox programs, or restrictive diets without scientific backing.

It's also essential to have open conversations with healthcare providers. Many patients are hesitant to discuss alternative treatments with their doctors, but a qualified medical professional can provide valuable insight into why certain treatments are ineffective or even harmful.

Conclusion

In conclusion, Reactive Hypoglycemia is a complex condition that requires careful dietary and lifestyle management. While the internet offers an abundance of information, not all of it is reliable or safe. Quack treatments, such as extreme diets, detox programs, and unregulated supplements, prey on the fears and vulnerabilities of patients, offering false hope in place of proven management strategies.

As patients continue their journey with Reactive Hypoglycemia, it is crucial to prioritize treatments that are backed by science and to remain vigilant against the dangers of quackery. By empowering themselves with knowledge and critical thinking skills, patients can make informed decisions about their health and avoid the pitfalls of pseudoscience.

2 The Rise of Quackery

Quackery is an age-old phenomenon that refers to the promotion and sale of fraudulent medical treatments and cures. The term "quack" describes someone who falsely claims to have medical knowledge or sells unproven and often harmful treatments. Over the centuries, quackery has taken many forms, from "miracle" elixirs to bizarre dietary practices, with countless people falling victim to false promises of healing. For Reactive Hypoglycemia patients, quack treatments present a particular danger because of the often confusing nature of their condition and the desperation they feel when conventional treatments fail to alleviate their symptoms or are not readily available. Understanding the history of quackery helps shed light on why such treatments are appealing to patients today and why vigilance is necessary to protect vulnerable populations.

Where Does the Name "Quack" Come From?

The word "quack" is derived from the Dutch word "quacksalver," which translates to "hawker of salve" or "peddler of ointments." In medieval Europe, "quacksalvers" were street vendors who sold homemade remedies, often loudly advertising their supposed healing powers in markets and public squares. These salesmen were known for their exaggerated claims and charismatic presentations, attracting large crowds with the promise of miracle cures. Over time, the term "quack" became synonymous with fraud, especially in the medical field, as many of these peddlers had no legitimate medical knowledge and sold treatments that were ineffective or even dangerous.

Quacks thrived during periods when medical knowledge was limited, and access to trained physicians was scarce. Before the advent of modern medicine, people relied on whatever treatment options were available, no matter how dubious. In the absence of proper medical regulations, quackery flourished. Quacks exploited the fear and desperation of those suffering from chronic or incurable illnesses, convincing them that their treatments could work where conventional medicine had failed. Even as science and medicine advanced, quackery evolved to keep up, adapting its methods and promises to fit new diseases and conditions.

Worst Quack Remedies in History

Throughout history, some of the worst quack remedies have gained widespread acceptance, often with disastrous consequences for patients. These remedies ranged from dangerous dietary practices to toxic tonics and outlandish contraptions. Here are some infamous examples:

1. **Radium Water** – In the early 20th century, radium, a radioactive element, was promoted as a miracle cure for everything from fatigue to digestive disorders. Radium water was sold as a tonic that would "recharge" the body with energy. Tragically, it caused radiation poisoning in those who drank it, leading to severe illness and death. One famous case involved Eben Byers, a wealthy industrialist who consumed large quantities of radium water and died from radiation poisoning, losing parts of his jaw and suffering excruciating pain before his death in 1932.

2. **Bloodletting** – For centuries, bloodletting was a common medical practice used to treat a variety of ailments, including infections and metabolic disorders. Physicians believed that removing blood from the body could balance the "humors" (bodily fluids thought to govern health).

This dangerous practice persisted for hundreds of years despite its lack of efficacy, often leaving patients weaker or leading to their death due to excessive blood loss.

3. **Snake Oil** – The term "snake oil" is now used as a metaphor for fraudulent health products, but in the 19th century, it referred to actual snake oil sold by quacks as a cure-all. Peddlers would claim their snake oil could treat everything from joint pain to digestive issues. In reality, these products often contained little or no actual snake oil and were usually composed of mineral oil, turpentine, and other cheap ingredients. The rise of snake oil salesmen gave birth to the modern connotation of "snake oil" as a deceptive remedy.

4. **Mercury and Arsenic Cures** – In the 18th and 19th centuries, mercury and arsenic were common ingredients in many "cures" for conditions such as diabetes or digestive problems. These toxic substances were believed to have healing properties but caused severe poisoning. Patients who took these treatments often suffered from neurological damage, organ failure, and death. Despite these well-known side effects, these remedies were widely accepted due to a lack of better alternatives.

5. **Dr. John Brinkley's Goat Gland Surgery** – One of the most bizarre examples of quackery in the 20th century was Dr. John Brinkley's "goat gland surgery." In the 1920s, Brinkley claimed he could cure male impotence by surgically implanting goat testicles into men. Despite having no medical training and no scientific basis for his procedure, Brinkley became wealthy and famous, performing thousands of surgeries. His procedures led to numerous deaths and lawsuits, and eventually, his medical license was revoked.

These treatments were accepted because they played on the fears and hopes of the sick. In many cases, people turned to quacks because conventional medicine either couldn't cure them or was inaccessible due to cost or geographic location. Quacks offered hope, even if it was false hope, and in desperate situations, people are often willing to try anything that might bring relief.

The Discovery of Reactive Hypoglycemia and Early Quackery

Reactive Hypoglycemia was first described in the early 20th century as a condition where the body experiences a rapid drop in blood sugar levels after eating, often leading to symptoms like dizziness, fatigue, and anxiety. Although Reactive Hypoglycemia is better understood today, early treatments were limited, and many patients were misdiagnosed or left untreated due to the lack of understanding around blood sugar regulation.

In the early 20th century, before the development of blood glucose monitoring, patients with Reactive Hypoglycemia might have been subjected to treatments like extreme diets or dangerous supplements claiming to "balance blood sugar." The condition's often vague symptoms made it a target for quacks who promised quick fixes, such as supplements or dietary regimens, to "cure" the body's inability to regulate glucose.

Why Reactive Hypoglycemia Patients Are Desperate for Quack Remedies

Today, patients with Reactive Hypoglycemia are still vulnerable to quack treatments, despite the availability of advanced medical knowledge and treatments. Reactive Hypoglycemia is a condition that can cause significant discomfort and daily disruptions. When conventional treatments, such as dietary adjustments, fail to provide complete relief, patients may feel compelled to explore alternative therapies.

The desperation Reactive Hypoglycemia patients feel is compounded by several factors:

1. **Chronic Symptoms** – Reactive Hypoglycemia can cause frequent fatigue, dizziness, and other symptoms that greatly diminish a patient's quality of life. When conventional treatments fail to provide relief, patients may feel they have no choice but to explore alternative

therapies.

2. **Uncertainty and Lack of Awareness** – Although Reactive Hypoglycemia is better understood today than in the past, there is still a lack of widespread awareness about the condition. Many patients struggle to find doctors familiar with Reactive Hypoglycemia, leading them to alternative practitioners who claim to have "cures."

3. **Long Wait Times for Treatment** – In some healthcare systems, patients face long wait times for diagnostic tests or treatment plans. This delay in receiving care can lead patients to seek quicker alternatives, even if those alternatives lack scientific support.

4. **False Promises of a Cure** – Quacks often exploit patients' desperation by offering false promises of a cure. While Reactive Hypoglycemia can be managed with proper diet and treatment, it cannot be "cured" by detox programs, supplements, or unregulated therapies. For patients seeking relief, these promises can be difficult to resist.

5. **Online Misinformation** – The internet has made it easier for quacks to reach vulnerable patients. Reactive Hypoglycemia patients can find countless websites, videos, and social media posts promoting unproven treatments, such as extreme diets or questionable supplements that may worsen symptoms or delay proper medical care.

Conclusion: The Continued Threat of Quackery

Quackery is as old as medicine itself, and despite advancements in medical science, it continues to pose a threat to patients, particularly those with conditions like Reactive Hypoglycemia. The history of quackery is a testament to the dangers of false hope and the importance of evidence-based medicine. From the street peddlers of medieval Europe to modern-day internet "gurus," quacks have preyed on the sick and vulnerable, offering fraudulent cures that often do more harm than good.

3 Dangerous Adjustments

Chiropractic treatment is a popular alternative therapy often used to address musculoskeletal problems like back pain, neck pain, and joint stiffness. Chiropractors focus on the alignment of the spine and believe that spinal adjustments can relieve pressure, restore mobility, and even treat a wide range of conditions, not all of which are musculoskeletal in nature. However, when it comes to metabolic conditions like Reactive Hypoglycemia (RH), chiropractic care enters dangerous territory.

Reactive Hypoglycemia is a condition characterized by episodes of low blood sugar that occur after meals, leading to symptoms such as dizziness, fatigue, weakness, and confusion. Some chiropractic practitioners claim that spinal adjustments can regulate blood sugar levels or even cure RH, despite no scientific evidence to support these claims. In fact, chiropractic manipulations can pose significant risks to RH patients, as this condition involves metabolic regulation, not spinal alignment. This chapter will explore the dangers of chiropractic care for RH patients, present real-life cautionary stories, and examine the controversies surrounding chiropractic adjustments.

Chiropractic Adjustments and Reactive Hypoglycemia: A Misguided Approach

Reactive Hypoglycemia is a metabolic disorder that primarily affects the body's ability to regulate blood sugar following meals. The causes of RH are varied, ranging from abnormal insulin response to underlying medical conditions like pre-diabetes or hormone imbalances. Chiropractors, however, may suggest that spinal misalignment is somehow contributing to this metabolic dysfunction, claiming that adjusting the spine can "reset" the body's blood sugar regulation.

Spinal adjustments, particularly those targeting the upper spine or neck, are based on the idea that correcting misalignments can improve overall health. But these adjustments do not address the underlying cause of Reactive Hypoglycemia—irregular glucose metabolism. Consequently, chiropractic care offers no legitimate solution for blood sugar regulation or the management of RH symptoms.

Patients with Reactive Hypoglycemia often require careful dietary planning, medical monitoring, and sometimes medications to manage their blood sugar. Chiropractic adjustments, on the other hand, are not only ineffective but can also distract patients from receiving proper care. In some cases, chiropractors may recommend dietary supplements or extreme diets, which can exacerbate the symptoms of RH, leading to dangerous fluctuations in blood sugar levels.

Patient Stories: The Dangers of Misinformation in Chiropractic Treatment

Patient stories provide real-world insights into the risks associated with inappropriate chiropractic treatment for metabolic disorders like Reactive Hypoglycemia. One alarming case involved a 45-year-old man who sought chiropractic care after experiencing fatigue, dizziness, and brain fog—a common symptom of RH. The chiropractor performed weekly spinal adjustments for two months, claiming that these treatments would help "balance" the patient's blood sugar.

Instead of improving, the patient's symptoms worsened. His blood sugar levels became more erratic, leading to episodes of severe hypoglycemia. At one point, he collapsed after a meal due to a drastic drop in blood sugar and was rushed to the emergency room, where he was finally diagnosed with Reactive Hypoglycemia. The delay in receiving proper medical care allowed the condition to worsen, and the patient had to undergo significant dietary and medical interventions to regain stability.

This patient's story highlights the dangers of relying on chiropractic care for a condition like RH. In this case, the chiropractor's failure to refer the patient to a medical professional who could properly diagnose and manage his condition led to serious complications.

Another case involved a young woman with RH who was advised by a chiropractor to take a variety of dietary supplements along with weekly spinal adjustments. The chiropractor claimed that these treatments would stabilize her blood sugar levels and cure her condition. Unfortunately, the combination of the supplements and unregulated diet exacerbated her symptoms, leading to episodes of extreme fatigue and confusion. It was later discovered that one of the supplements interfered with her prescribed medication, worsening her hypoglycemia and delaying effective treatment.

These stories serve as cautionary examples of how chiropractic care, when applied inappropriately to conditions like RH, can result in delayed diagnosis, worsening symptoms, and harmful interactions with necessary medical treatments.

The History and Controversies of Chiropractic Adjustments

Chiropractic care was founded by Daniel David Palmer in the late 19th century. Palmer believed that spinal misalignments, which he called "subluxations," were the root cause of many health problems. He theorized that by adjusting the spine, chiropractors could correct these subluxations and restore the body's natural ability to heal itself. While chiropractic care has gained mainstream acceptance for treating musculoskeletal issues, it remains controversial, particularly when it claims to treat non-musculoskeletal conditions like Reactive Hypoglycemia.

One of the most contentious aspects of chiropractic care is

the lack of scientific evidence supporting the subluxation theory. Numerous studies have failed to demonstrate any measurable health benefits from chiropractic adjustments beyond temporary relief from pain. When it comes to metabolic conditions like RH, the idea that spinal adjustments could affect blood sugar regulation is not only unsupported by evidence but also dangerously misleading.

For patients with Reactive Hypoglycemia, a metabolic disorder that requires careful management through diet and medical care, chiropractic adjustments offer no real benefit. Chiropractors who claim they can treat or cure RH through spinal manipulation are engaging in medical misinformation, putting patients at risk by delaying necessary care.

The Risk of Misinformation in Chiropractic Care

One of the biggest challenges for patients seeking chiropractic care is distinguishing between reputable practitioners who focus on musculoskeletal issues and those who make exaggerated claims about treating a wide range of conditions. The chiropractic field is not as rigorously regulated as conventional medicine, leading to significant variability in the quality of care.

For patients with Reactive Hypoglycemia, this lack of regulation can be especially dangerous. Chiropractors who promote unproven treatments for RH, such as spinal adjustments or dietary supplements, may inadvertently cause harm by preventing patients from receiving evidence-based care from qualified medical professionals. In some cases, patients are advised to adopt extreme diets or take supplements that may interfere with their medication or worsen their condition, further complicating the management of their blood sugar levels.

Chiropractic Care vs. Medical Care: Why RH Requires Proper Treatment

For patients with Reactive Hypoglycemia, proper medical care is essential. Effective management of RH involves identifying the underlying cause of the condition, making appropriate dietary changes, and, in some cases, using medications to regulate blood sugar levels. Unlike chiropractic adjustments, which focus on spinal alignment, medical treatment for RH addresses the actual metabolic dysfunction responsible for hypoglycemic episodes.

Chiropractors who claim they can treat or cure Reactive Hypoglycemia through spinal adjustments are not only misleading their patients but also putting them at risk of delayed or improper treatment. For patients with severe symptoms, the delay in receiving appropriate medical care can lead to serious complications, including the development of more severe metabolic disorders.

Conclusion: Chiropractic Adjustments Are Not a Cure for Reactive Hypoglycemia

In conclusion, while chiropractic care may be helpful for managing musculoskeletal pain, it is not an appropriate or effective treatment for Reactive Hypoglycemia. The metabolic issues that define RH cannot be corrected by spinal adjustments, and any claim to the contrary is misleading and potentially harmful. Patient stories like those shared in this chapter demonstrate the risks of chiropractic care for RH patients, from worsening symptoms to delayed diagnosis.

For patients with Reactive Hypoglycemia, the best course of action is to seek care from medical professionals who specialize in metabolic conditions. Chiropractic adjustments, particularly when paired with unregulated supplements or extreme dietary advice, should be avoided due to the risks of further complications. Proper medical care—not pseudoscientific treatments—is the key to managing RH and preventing long-term health issues.

4 Beware Cranial Therapy

Cranial therapy, also known as Craniosacral Therapy (CST), is a pseudoscientific practice often promoted by alternative medicine practitioners as a treatment for a wide array of health conditions, including Reactive Hypoglycemia (RH). Despite lacking credible scientific evidence, some quacks recommend this therapy for managing RH, exploiting patients' desperation for relief from the often disruptive symptoms of this condition. This chapter will explore what cranial therapy entails, why it is dangerous, how it differs from chiropractic adjustments, and the underlying reasons it is recommended by unscrupulous practitioners.

What is Cranial Therapy?

Cranial therapy is based on a series of false premises. Proponents of CST claim that the human brain makes rhythmic movements, independent of heartbeats or respiration, at a rate of 10 to 14 cycles per minute. According to them, these movements create a "craniosacral rhythm," which can be detected by a practitioner's fingertips. They also assert that small pulsations in the skull bones—where the cranial sutures meet—affect the flow of cerebrospinal fluid (CSF) and that diseases are caused by disturbances in this rhythm.

Cranial therapists claim that applying gentle pressure to the skull can release restrictions, restore CSF flow, and treat conditions like Reactive Hypoglycemia. Despite these extraordinary claims, there is no scientific evidence to support the existence of the craniosacral rhythm or that manipulating the skull bones can cure any disease. In fact, the skull bones are fused by adolescence, making it impossible to manipulate them in the way CST practitioners claim.

Why Cranial Therapy is Recommended by Quacks

The recommendation of cranial therapy by quacks often stems from the desperation of patients suffering from conditions like Reactive Hypoglycemia, where conventional treatments may offer only partial relief, or dietary adjustments may be challenging. These patients are often searching for alternative treatments that seem less invasive or more holistic than traditional medical interventions.

Quacks take advantage of this desperation by promoting CST as a "gentle" and "noninvasive" alternative to medical treatments. They often make sweeping claims that CST can improve overall health, stabilize blood sugar levels, and alleviate conditions ranging from headaches to metabolic disorders like RH. For someone struggling with blood sugar crashes and the fatigue and confusion of RH, the appeal of a natural, noninvasive therapy can be strong.

The Upledger Institute, a major promoter of CST, has even suggested that CST can relieve conditions as varied as chronic fatigue, autism, and digestive issues. Practitioners claim that realigning the craniosacral system can address numerous health problems, but these assertions are not grounded in scientific reality.

Why Cranial Therapy is Dangerous

For patients with Reactive Hypoglycemia, cranial therapy poses significant risks. RH is a metabolic condition that results from an abnormal insulin response to food, causing blood sugar levels to drop too low. The idea that gentle pressure on the skull could stabilize blood sugar or affect the body's metabolic processes is not only false but potentially harmful.

One of the primary dangers of cranial therapy is that it may delay or replace legitimate medical treatment. Managing RH requires careful dietary planning, possibly medications, and regular monitoring of blood sugar levels. By opting for CST instead of evidence-based medical treatments, patients risk allowing their condition to worsen. Hypoglycemic episodes can lead to fainting, seizures, or even coma if left untreated.

Though CST practitioners claim that their manipulations are gentle—using no more than five grams of pressure—this manipulation offers no real benefit for metabolic disorders like RH. The lack of proper medical care or nutritional guidance can exacerbate RH symptoms, leading to dangerous consequences.

Reported Dangers and Deaths

Several cases have highlighted the dangers of cranial therapy, particularly when it is used as a substitute for proper medical care. Though specific reports linking CST directly to RH are scarce, broader examples demonstrate the risks of this pseudoscientific practice. For instance, in one case, a chiropractor advised a woman with epilepsy to stop her medication in favor of cranial therapy. She later died from severe seizures. Another case involved a dentist performing CST on an infant with a high fever, resulting in the infant's death due to complications from skull manipulation.

These cases demonstrate the irresponsibility of some cranial therapists and their disregard for scientific medical practices. While such extreme outcomes are not common, they emphasize the real risks associated with relying on pseudoscience instead of proven treatments.

The Difference Between Cranial Therapy and Chiropractic Adjustments

Cranial therapy and chiropractic adjustments may seem similar because both involve physical manipulation of the body, but they differ significantly in their methods and claims. Chiropractic care focuses on the alignment of the spine, with chiropractors believing that misalignments (subluxations) interfere with nerve function. Chiropractic adjustments may help relieve musculoskeletal pain, but the practice becomes controversial when applied to non-musculoskeletal conditions.

Cranial therapy, however, focuses on manipulating the bones of the skull and claims to affect the flow of cerebrospinal fluid, a premise rejected by mainstream medicine. CST practitioners claim to feel and correct craniosacral rhythms, which have no recognition in legitimate medical fields. Though some chiropractors incorporate cranial manipulation into their practices, the two treatments are based on different pseudoscientific principles.

The major distinction lies in the focus—chiropractic adjustments target the spine, while CST targets the skull. Both practices lack evidence when applied to conditions like Reactive Hypoglycemia, but CST is particularly dangerous because it addresses a condition that is metabolic in nature, not structural.

The Scientific Perspective on Cranial Therapy

The scientific community has consistently rejected cranial therapy as a valid treatment. Several studies have concluded that the fundamental premise of CST—the existence of craniosacral rhythms and the ability to manipulate them—lacks any scientific basis. The British Columbia Office of Health Technology Assessment reviewed the evidence for CST and concluded that "there is insufficient evidence to recommend craniosacral therapy to patients, practitioners, or third-party payers."

Moreover, attempts to measure the so-called craniosacral rhythms have been inconsistent. In one study, different therapists examining the same patients reported significantly different measurements of the craniosacral rate. This inconsistency further undermines the credibility of CST as a legitimate practice.

Additionally, anatomical studies show that the cranial bones fuse during adolescence, making it impossible for them to move as CST practitioners claim. The idea that manipulating these bones can treat metabolic disorders like RH is pure fantasy.

How Patients Can Identify Pseudoscientific Practices

For patients with Reactive Hypoglycemia, it is essential to distinguish between evidence-based treatments and pseudoscientific practices like cranial therapy. One key indicator of a legitimate treatment is whether it is supported by peer-reviewed research published in reputable medical journals.

Patients can check if a journal is peer-reviewed by researching its publication process. Peer-reviewed journals require that articles be evaluated by experts in the field before publication, ensuring that the research is credible and based on sound methodology.

Some reputable peer-reviewed journals that cover dietary and metabolic interventions include:

1. The Journal of Clinical Endocrinology & Metabolism

2. Diabetes Care

3. The Lancet

4. The New England Journal of Medicine

5. JAMA: The Journal of the American Medical Association

Patients should be cautious of treatments not backed by research published in such journals.

Conclusion

Cranial therapy is a dangerous pseudoscientific practice that preys on vulnerable patients, offering false hope for conditions like Reactive Hypoglycemia. The premise that manipulating the skull can treat metabolic conditions is not supported by any credible scientific evidence. For patients with RH, choosing CST over legitimate medical treatments can lead to worsened symptoms and, in some cases, irreversible harm. It is essential to seek evidence-based treatments and consult healthcare providers who rely on scientific research rather than pseudoscientific practices.

Reference:

Barrett, Stephen. "Why Cranial Therapy Is Silly." *Quackwatch*, 15 May 2004, https://quackwatch.org/related/dental-education/hcra/cranial. Accessed 24 Oct. 2024.

5 The Vegan Diet Myth

In the realm of alternative health, using diet to manage various conditions has gained significant traction. One of the more extreme claims is the idea that adopting a vegan or raw vegan diet can cure or significantly improve conditions like Reactive Hypoglycemia (RH). While plant-based diets offer well-documented health benefits, particularly in managing cardiovascular health, reducing inflammation, and improving general wellness, the assertion that such diets can cure RH is misleading. This chapter explores the false claims surrounding vegan diets and their purported effects on RH, while highlighting the legitimate benefits of plant-based eating for overall health.

The Appeal of Vegan and Raw Vegan Diets

The appeal of veganism, especially raw veganism, lies in its focus on natural, whole foods that are free from processed ingredients and animal products. Proponents argue that such a diet can reduce inflammation, lower the risk of chronic diseases like heart disease and diabetes, and promote overall well-being. While these claims are generally true when it comes to general health, they are not a cure for Reactive Hypoglycemia.

For individuals with RH, the allure of such diets is based on the misleading belief that veganism can stabilize blood sugar levels and alleviate the condition's metabolic symptoms. Many alternative health practitioners argue that eating plant-based can "reset" the body and resolve the blood sugar fluctuations that characterize RH. However, this is a gross oversimplification of the metabolic disorder.

False Claims Surrounding Vegan Diets and Reactive Hypoglycemia

Reactive Hypoglycemia is a condition where the body experiences abnormally low blood sugar after eating, often in response to carbohydrate-heavy meals. Proponents of vegan diets claim that cutting out animal products and processed foods can improve insulin sensitivity and regulate blood sugar. While plant-based diets rich in fiber, whole grains, and low-glycemic foods may help regulate glucose levels to some extent, they cannot "cure" RH.

One of the most common arguments from vegan diet advocates is that inflammation plays a role in metabolic disorders and that adopting a vegan diet can reduce inflammation to the point of alleviating RH symptoms. However, RH's symptoms are primarily driven by hormonal and metabolic responses that cannot be resolved by simply eliminating animal products. Blood sugar regulation requires a balanced approach to managing carbohydrate intake, protein, and fats—none of which can be adequately addressed by a restrictive diet alone.

Patient Desperation and the Appeal of Dietary Cures

For many people suffering from Reactive Hypoglycemia, the persistent symptoms of blood sugar fluctuations—dizziness, shakiness, weakness, and confusion—lead to desperation. When conventional dietary approaches or medications don't offer immediate relief, patients may turn to vegan or raw vegan diets, hoping for an alternative solution.

It's understandable that individuals with RH might be drawn to such diets, as they promote health and wellness while offering an attractive "natural" solution. However, no amount of dietary modification can change the fact that RH is a metabolic issue that requires medical management. The body's ability to process and regulate glucose involves complex hormonal pathways, and relying on diet alone, especially without professional guidance, can lead to dangerous blood sugar lows.

The Legitimate Health Benefits of a Vegan Diet

Although vegan diets cannot cure RH, it's important to acknowledge the substantial health benefits that plant-based eating can offer. Vegan diets are rich in anti-inflammatory foods, such as leafy greens, berries, and whole grains, which can help reduce systemic inflammation. For those managing the discomfort that comes with fluctuating energy levels or mild fatigue, these anti-inflammatory foods can help improve overall well-being.

Additionally, vegan diets tend to be lower in saturated fats and cholesterol, improving cardiovascular health and potentially benefiting those with secondary health concerns like high blood pressure. Plant-based diets are also associated with better weight management, which may indirectly benefit people with RH by promoting overall metabolic health.

The Risk of Poorly Planned Vegan Diets and Nutritional Deficiencies in RH

One of the significant risks of adopting a poorly planned vegan diet is the potential for nutritional deficiencies, which can be especially problematic for individuals with Reactive Hypoglycemia. RH patients must carefully balance their intake of carbohydrates, protein, and fats to avoid triggering hypoglycemic episodes. A vegan diet that lacks sufficient protein or healthy fats may exacerbate blood sugar issues rather than alleviate them.

Moreover, certain nutrients like vitamin B12, iron, calcium, and omega-3 fatty acids can be deficient in a vegan diet if not properly supplemented. For those with RH, these deficiencies can lead to fatigue, weakness, and further metabolic complications. Vitamin B12, in particular, is crucial for maintaining healthy energy levels and neurological function, and without it, RH symptoms may worsen.

Case Study: Vitamin B12 Deficiency in an RH Patient

A case study from **BMJ Case Reports** illustrates the dangers of vitamin B12 deficiency in a patient with Reactive

Hypoglycemia. The patient, a long-term vegan, presented with severe fatigue, muscle weakness, and hypoglycemic episodes. Upon further examination, the patient's vitamin B12 levels were found to be dangerously low, leading to neurological symptoms and worsening blood sugar control.

After receiving vitamin B12 supplementation, the patient's energy levels and blood sugar regulation significantly improved, highlighting the importance of proper nutrient intake in managing RH. This case underscores the risks of adopting extreme diets without adequate nutritional support, particularly for patients dealing with complex metabolic conditions like Reactive Hypoglycemia.

Can a Vegan Diet Help Manage RH Symptoms?

While a vegan diet cannot cure Reactive Hypoglycemia, it may help manage some symptoms, particularly if the diet includes balanced macronutrient intake and is rich in low-glycemic foods. Plant-based diets that emphasize whole grains, legumes, and nuts can provide steady, slow-releasing carbohydrates that may help regulate blood sugar levels.

However, it is crucial to ensure that vegan diets for RH patients are carefully planned to avoid deficiencies in protein and healthy fats, both of which are essential for maintaining stable blood sugar levels. Consulting with a healthcare provider or dietitian can help ensure that a vegan diet is tailored to meet the specific nutritional needs of individuals with RH.

Conclusion: A Balanced Approach to Diet and Health for RH Patients

In conclusion, while a vegan or raw vegan diet cannot cure Reactive Hypoglycemia, adopting a well-balanced, plant-based diet can offer significant health benefits. These include reducing inflammation, promoting cardiovascular health, and improving mental well-being, all of which can indirectly help manage some of the symptoms associated with RH. However, it's essential to approach dietary changes with caution, especially in the context of a condition like Reactive Hypoglycemia, where blood sugar regulation is key.

RH patients should be wary of extreme dietary claims that promise a cure, and instead focus on evidence-based dietary approaches. Consulting with a nutritionist or healthcare provider ensures that dietary changes support rather than hinder health, allowing patients to manage their condition effectively while maintaining proper nutrient intake. By adopting a balanced, well-planned diet, individuals with RH can enjoy the benefits of plant-based eating while avoiding the risks of nutritional deficiencies.

6 Other Pseudoscientific Diets

The alkaline diet is based on the belief that certain foods can alter the acidity or alkalinity (pH) of the body's fluids, particularly the blood, and that consuming more alkaline foods can help prevent or even reverse diseases. Proponents of this diet claim that it can alleviate a variety of conditions, including Reactive Hypoglycemia (RH). However, this notion is grounded in pseudoscience and is not supported by any credible evidence in the medical literature. While a diet rich in fruits and vegetables can improve overall health, there is no scientifically sound evidence to suggest that it can cure or alleviate the symptoms of RH, which is a complex metabolic condition related to blood sugar regulation.

In addition to the alkaline diet, other pseudoscientific diets make false claims about curing or managing conditions like RH. The raw food diet, for example, is often promoted as a way to "detox" the body and heal chronic conditions, but no scientific evidence supports the idea that eating only raw foods can cure metabolic or neurological issues. Another extreme is the carnivore diet, which advocates for eating only meat and animal products. Proponents claim it can reduce inflammation and balance blood sugar, but no credible medical literature supports these assertions. Other fad diets, such as juice cleanses or prolonged fasting regimens, promise to "reset" the body's blood sugar system but lack scientific validity and can lead to dangerous nutrient deficiencies.

These diets, like the alkaline diet, mislead patients by promoting radical dietary changes as a cure for serious conditions. This chapter will explore the pseudoscientific foundation of the alkaline diet, discuss how credibility is determined in medical research, and explain how patients can ensure that the diets they choose are based on sound science.

The Alkaline Diet: Misunderstanding Human Physiology

The core premise of the alkaline diet is that certain foods can change the pH of the body and make it less acidic. Advocates claim that a more alkaline environment in the body can prevent or even cure various diseases, including cancer, arthritis, and conditions like Reactive Hypoglycemia. However, this claim ignores fundamental aspects of human physiology.

The human body tightly regulates its pH levels, especially in the blood, where the normal pH ranges from 7.35 to 7.45. The body maintains this balance through various mechanisms, such as kidney function and respiratory control, which ensure that blood pH remains stable. These mechanisms are vital for survival, and no amount of dietary change can significantly alter blood pH in a healthy person. If the body's pH were to shift outside this narrow range, it would indicate a serious medical condition, such as acidosis or alkalosis, which requires immediate medical attention—not a dietary intervention.

While certain foods can temporarily alter the pH of urine, this does not reflect a change in the body's overall pH balance. This change is part of the body's natural process to regulate blood pH. The idea that diet alone can "balance" the body's pH and resolve conditions like Reactive Hypoglycemia is not only incorrect but also potentially harmful.

Lack of Credible Support: What It Really Means

The alkaline diet, like many other pseudoscientific health fads, lacks credible support in the medical literature. But what exactly does "credible" mean in this context? Understanding how scientific credibility is measured is essential to recognizing valid claims versus pseudoscientific ones.

In the medical and scientific communities, credibility is determined by several factors:

1. **Peer Review Process**: Credible studies are published in peer-reviewed journals, where independent experts in the field assess the study's methodology, data, and conclusions to ensure they are sound and unbiased. This vetting process is designed to catch errors and prevent bias. If a claim, such as the alkaline diet's ability to cure RH, is not supported by peer-reviewed research, it should be viewed with skepticism.

2. **Reproducibility of Results**: For research to be considered credible, its results must be reproducible. This means that other researchers should be able to conduct the same experiment and achieve similar results. If a dietary claim is based on a single study or anecdotal evidence and cannot be replicated, it is not considered reliable.

3. **Sample Size and Control Groups**: Credible research involves sufficiently large sample sizes and includes control groups to ensure that the findings are not due to chance or other factors. Many of the studies promoting diets like the alkaline diet lack control groups or have very small sample sizes, which undermines their credibility.

4. **Absence of Bias**: Scientific credibility also depends on the absence of financial or personal bias. Studies funded by companies with vested interests in selling supplements or diet plans may be biased toward favorable results. Credible research is transparent about its funding sources and potential conflicts of interest.

5. **Plausibility Based on Established Science**: For a new claim to be credible, it must make sense in the context of existing scientific knowledge. The premise of the alkaline diet—that foods can significantly alter blood pH and affect disease outcomes—is implausible based on established knowledge of human physiology and biochemistry.

How to Identify Peer-Reviewed Research

For patients unfamiliar with scientific research, identifying credible sources can be challenging. However, there are ways to ensure that the information being considered has scientific backing:

1. **Look for Peer-Reviewed Journals**: Peer-reviewed journals are the gold standard for reliable scientific information. Journals like *The New England Journal of Medicine*, *The Lancet*, and *The Journal of Nutrition* only publish studies reviewed by experts in the field. Databases like PubMed index research from reputable, peer-reviewed sources.

2. **Consult Meta-Analyses and Systematic Reviews**: These types of research synthesize the findings of multiple studies, offering a comprehensive overview. If a diet like the alkaline diet were effective, there would be multiple high-quality studies supporting it, which would be summarized in meta-analyses or systematic reviews.

3. **Watch Out for Red Flags**: Be skeptical of health claims based on anecdotal evidence, personal testimonials, or promises of a "miracle cure." Diets that claim to cure complex conditions like Reactive Hypoglycemia are likely too good to be true.

4. **Trusted Medical Sources**: Government health agencies such as the National Institutes of Health (NIH) and reputable organizations like the Mayo Clinic provide reliable, science-backed information on health and nutrition.

A List of Peer-Reviewed Journals on Diet and Nutrition

Here are a few reputable, peer-reviewed journals that regularly publish research on diet and nutrition:

- *The American Journal of Clinical Nutrition*
- *The Journal of Nutrition*

- *Nutrition Reviews*
- *The British Journal of Nutrition*
- *The Journal of the Academy of Nutrition and Dietetics*
- *Public Health Nutrition*
- *Nutrition and Metabolism*

These journals are reliable sources for accurate information on the health effects of various diets. If a diet is genuinely beneficial, supporting studies will be published in these types of journals.

Why Are Pseudoscientific Diets Like the Alkaline Diet So Popular?

Despite the lack of credible evidence, diets like the alkaline diet remain popular, especially among those with chronic conditions. Several factors contribute to their appeal:

1. **Desperation for Relief**: Patients with chronic illnesses like RH often experience persistent symptoms that conventional treatments cannot fully resolve. The promise of a dietary cure, even without scientific backing, can seem like a beacon of hope.

2. **Appeal of Natural Remedies**: Many pseudoscientific diets market themselves as "natural" solutions, which appeals to individuals wary of pharmaceuticals or medical interventions.

3. **Mistrust of Conventional Medicine**: Some patients turn to alternative diets because they feel that conventional medicine has failed them or because they mistrust the pharmaceutical industry.

4. **Persuasive Marketing**: The marketing behind pseudoscientific diets often uses emotional appeals and personal testimonials to attract patients, even though these claims lack scientific validation.

5. **Confirmation Bias**: Patients who adopt pseudoscientific

diets may attribute any improvement in their condition to the diet, even if the improvement is due to other lifestyle changes or a placebo effect.

Ensuring Credibility When Choosing a Diet

For patients with Reactive Hypoglycemia, it's essential to ensure that their dietary choices are supported by credible, peer-reviewed research. While a balanced diet can support overall health, it's important to avoid diets that make false claims about curing RH. By focusing on sound science and paying attention to credible research, patients can make informed decisions that promote long-term health without falling victim to pseudoscientific claims.

Conclusion

In conclusion, the alkaline diet and similar pseudoscientific diets fail to offer any credible solution for managing or curing Reactive Hypoglycemia. While the promotion of whole foods and a balanced diet is valuable for overall health, the claims that these diets can alter the body's pH and cure complex conditions like RH are false. Patients should rely on diets grounded in scientific evidence and steer clear of extreme or unproven dietary approaches. By focusing on balanced nutrition, supported by credible research, individuals with Reactive Hypoglycemia can manage their condition effectively and avoid the false hope offered by pseudoscientific diets.

7 Homeopathy: Diluting Reality

Homeopathy, despite being widely criticized and scientifically disproven, remains a popular alternative medicine system. It is based on two main principles: "like cures like" and extreme dilution. While many people turn to homeopathy for chronic conditions, it has no place in treating metabolic disorders like Reactive Hypoglycemia (RH).

Reactive Hypoglycemia involves sudden drops in blood sugar levels following meals, often resulting in symptoms such as dizziness, shakiness, weakness, and confusion. This is a condition rooted in the body's insulin response and glucose regulation, issues that cannot be addressed by homeopathic remedies diluted to the point of being essentially non-existent. Despite the lack of scientific support, some homeopaths claim that their remedies can manage or cure the symptoms of RH.

This chapter explores the foundations of homeopathy, explains why homeopathic treatments are ineffective for conditions like Reactive Hypoglycemia, and highlights patient stories that demonstrate the dangers of choosing homeopathy over evidence-based medical treatments.

The Appeal of Homeopathy for RH Patients

Homeopathy has maintained its popularity for over two centuries, even as modern medicine has advanced significantly. Part of its enduring appeal lies in its perceived safety—homeopathic remedies are often marketed as "natural," "gentle," and "free from side effects." Many individuals with chronic or poorly understood conditions, such as RH, may feel frustrated with conventional treatments, which require constant dietary monitoring, lifestyle changes, or medications that can have side effects. Homeopathy, with its promise of a simple, holistic cure, can appear to be a more attractive option.

Additionally, homeopathic practitioners tend to spend a significant amount of time with their patients, offering empathy, attention, and a personalized approach to care. This level of attention can stand in stark contrast to the sometimes rushed environment of conventional medicine, where patients with RH may see multiple specialists and face long waiting periods between appointments. The combination of personal attention, the promise of an easy cure, and frustration with conventional treatments can lead patients toward homeopathy, even when it is ineffective or potentially harmful.

The Dangers of Homeopathy for Reactive Hypoglycemia

While the appeal of homeopathy is understandable, the dangers are considerable. Reactive Hypoglycemia is a metabolic disorder involving glucose regulation, and homeopathy cannot address the underlying biological mechanisms that lead to these sudden blood sugar drops. Relying on homeopathy as a treatment for RH can result in serious consequences.

One of the primary dangers of homeopathy is the delay it causes in receiving appropriate medical care. For patients managing RH, consistent blood sugar regulation is critical. Failing to address the condition properly can lead to more severe hypoglycemic episodes, which could cause confusion, loss of consciousness, or other life-threatening complications. Patients who use homeopathic remedies in place of proven dietary or medical management risk exacerbating their condition.

Consider the case of Sarah, a 35-year-old RH patient who experienced frequent blood sugar crashes. Afraid of medications and frustrated with the constant need for dietary monitoring, she turned to homeopathy. A homeopath assured her that a series of diluted remedies could stabilize her blood sugar levels, and she began using these treatments. Over the next several months, Sarah's hypoglycemic episodes worsened, leading to a near-fatal incident where she fainted while driving. After being rushed to the hospital, her doctors informed her that delaying proper management had allowed her condition to become increasingly dangerous.

Sarah's story is not unique. Many patients with chronic conditions, including RH, turn to homeopathy in hopes of avoiding the challenges of conventional management or because they believe in the body's ability to heal itself. However, when it comes to a metabolic disorder like RH, there is no substitute for medical management, whether that involves dietary changes, medications, or continuous glucose monitoring.

Why Homeopathy Cannot Address RH's Biological Issues

Homeopathy is based on the idea that "like cures like"—the notion that a substance that causes symptoms in a healthy person can cure those same symptoms in a sick person when diluted to extreme levels. For example, a homeopath might suggest that a diluted solution of glucose could help manage blood sugar issues because glucose is what triggers RH episodes in high amounts. However, this principle does not hold up to scientific scrutiny. Homeopathic remedies are so diluted that they contain no active ingredients, and numerous studies have shown that they are no more effective than placebos.

Even if homeopathy could somehow trigger a healing response for minor ailments (which it does not), it would still be incapable of addressing the complex metabolic and biological processes involved in Reactive Hypoglycemia. The core problem in RH is an abnormal insulin response following meals, leading to sharp drops in blood sugar levels. No amount of diluted substances can alter insulin production or stabilize glucose levels.

Homeopathic practitioners may claim that their remedies can relieve RH symptoms like dizziness, weakness, or confusion, but these claims are unsupported by any credible evidence. While patients may experience temporary relief through the placebo effect, this does not address the underlying cause of their condition. Over time, as blood sugar continues to fluctuate, symptoms will inevitably return or worsen. Delaying effective treatment for RH can lead to severe complications, making reliance on homeopathy a dangerous gamble.

Guy Chapman's Critique of Homeopathy

Guy Chapman, in his critique of homeopathy presented to a U.K. Parliamentary Committee, emphasizes the dangers of homeopathy for serious medical conditions. His arguments are particularly relevant for patients with conditions like RH, as they highlight the risks of relying on pseudoscientific treatments that lack credible evidence.

Chapman draws attention to the frequent misrepresentation of sources by homeopaths. He cites the example of the "Health Technology Assessment" (HTA), which homeopaths presented as a legitimate study. However, Chapman reveals that this HTA was a biased and reworked version of a previously failed submission to the Swiss Government's complementary medicine evaluation program. This example illustrates how proponents of homeopathy may distort evidence to support their claims.

Chapman also references a meta-analysis published in *The Lancet*, which found no compelling evidence that homeopathy worked better than a placebo. He explains that studies showing positive results for homeopathy often have weak methodologies. The more rigorously a study is designed, the less likely it is to show any benefit from homeopathic treatments.

For patients with RH, Chapman's critique serves as a stark reminder that homeopathy cannot substitute for scientifically validated treatments. Using homeopathy to treat serious metabolic conditions like RH can delay proper medical intervention and worsen a patient's health.

Patient Stories: False Hope and Real Harm

In addition to Sarah's case, many other RH patients have turned to homeopathy only to be disappointed by the lack of results. Some have spent thousands of dollars on homeopathic treatments over several months or years, only to find themselves in worse condition than before.

Take the story of James, a 50-year-old man who had been managing RH for years. After hearing about homeopathy's supposed benefits for blood sugar regulation, he decided to try it, despite his doctor's warnings. Over the course of six months, James's homeopath prescribed a series of remedies, including diluted solutions of various plants and minerals. At first, James thought he felt better, but the placebo effect was likely at work. Eventually, his blood sugar crashes became so severe that he was admitted to the hospital with dangerously low glucose levels. His doctors informed him that his reliance on homeopathy had worsened his condition, making recovery more difficult.

James's story demonstrates the false hope that homeopathy offers. Patients are led to believe that they are receiving treatment, but in reality, they are using remedies that are nothing more than sugar pills and water. The time and money spent on homeopathy are wasted, and the patient's health continues to deteriorate while they pursue an impossible cure.

Conclusion: Diluting Reality

In conclusion, homeopathy is based on principles that have no scientific foundation. The U.S. National Center for Complementary and Integrative Health (NCCIH) states, "There is little evidence to support homeopathy as an effective treatment for any specific condition" and "several key concepts of homeopathy are inconsistent with fundamental concepts of chemistry and physics."

For conditions like Reactive Hypoglycemia, which involve complex metabolic processes and glucose regulation, homeopathic remedies are not just ineffective—they are dangerously misleading. The false hope they offer can delay effective medical treatment, leading to worsening symptoms and potentially life-threatening complications. While homeopathy may seem like a gentle, natural alternative to medications or dietary management, it is nothing more than a placebo. It has no place in the treatment of Reactive Hypoglycemia.

References:

Chapman, Guy. "Written Evidence Submitted by Guy Chapman (AMR0058)." *Parliament UK*, 17 Dec. 2012, https://committees.parliament.uk/writtenevidence/48855/html/.

National Center for Complementary and Integrative Health. "Homeopathy." *NCCIH*, U.S. Department of Health and Human Services, Aug. 2016, www.nccih.nih.gov/health/homeopathy.

8 Promises Without Proof

Energy healing, which includes practices like Reiki, Therapeutic Touch, and Qi Gong, is often marketed as a gentle, non-invasive method to relieve various ailments. Practitioners claim to balance or manipulate a person's "life energy" to promote healing. These therapies involve little to no physical contact and rely on the belief that the practitioner can direct healing energy into or around the patient's body. For individuals suffering from chronic conditions such as Reactive Hypoglycemia (RH), energy healing is sometimes suggested as a way to alleviate symptoms like fatigue, dizziness, and confusion. However, despite its appeal as a natural and non-invasive option, energy healing lacks scientific support and poses dangers for those with serious health conditions like RH.

This chapter delves into the pseudoscientific foundations of energy healing practices, including Reiki, and explains why they are ineffective for managing conditions like RH. We'll explore the difference between patient testimonials and clinical outcomes, the risks posed by these therapies for those with complex metabolic disorders, and how the placebo effect plays a significant role in any perceived benefits.

The Pseudoscientific Foundation of Energy Healing

Energy healing is based on the belief that an invisible "life energy" or "vital energy" flows through and around the human body. In different cultures, this energy is known by various names: qi in Chinese medicine, prana in Hinduism, and ki in Reiki. Energy healers claim that disruptions or imbalances in this energy can lead to illness and that by manipulating or directing the energy, they can restore balance and alleviate symptoms.

Reiki, one of the most well-known forms of energy healing, was developed in Japan in the early 20th century by Mikao Usui. Reiki practitioners claim to channel energy from a universal source into the patient, promoting healing and well-being. Today, Reiki is often advertised as a way to relieve stress, improve general health, and, in some cases, treat conditions like Reactive Hypoglycemia.

Despite these claims, there is no scientific evidence supporting the existence of "life energy" or that energy healing can influence health. The human body does not contain measurable energy fields that can be manipulated to promote healing. The principles behind energy healing contradict established scientific understanding of biology and physics, making these practices pseudoscientific.

Testimonials Versus Clinical Outcomes

Energy healing continues to be popular, largely due to the numerous patient testimonials that report relief after sessions. Patients often describe feeling more relaxed, less stressed, or even experience reduced symptoms like fatigue or dizziness after energy healing treatments. While these testimonials can be compelling, they are anecdotal and subjective, and they do not constitute scientific proof of effectiveness.

Anecdotal evidence is unreliable because it is influenced by numerous factors, including placebo effects, natural symptom fluctuations, and personal biases. Patients may attribute their improvement to energy healing when, in reality, other factors such as natural recovery, lifestyle changes, or the passage of time may have contributed to their relief.

In contrast, the effectiveness of a treatment is determined

through rigorous scientific methods, such as randomized controlled trials (RCTs). To date, no high-quality clinical studies have demonstrated that energy healing practices like Reiki offer any benefits beyond placebo. Any improvement that patients report can typically be explained by the placebo effect, rather than by any real manipulation of life energy.

Why Energy Healing Is Dangerous for Patients with Reactive Hypoglycemia

For patients with Reactive Hypoglycemia, relying on energy healing can be particularly dangerous. RH is a metabolic disorder involving abnormal insulin responses that cause blood sugar levels to drop dramatically after eating, leading to symptoms like shakiness, dizziness, fatigue, and even fainting. Managing RH requires careful dietary planning, regular monitoring, and sometimes medical intervention. Energy healing cannot regulate insulin production or stabilize glucose levels, making it ineffective for addressing the root causes of RH.

One significant risk of energy healing is that it may give patients a false sense of security. Believing their symptoms are improving due to Reiki or another energy healing practice, RH patients may delay seeking medical care or making necessary lifestyle changes. This delay can result in more frequent or severe hypoglycemic episodes, putting their health at risk.

Additionally, the field of energy healing is largely unregulated, meaning practitioners are not required to have medical training or certifications in most areas. This lack of regulation leaves patients vulnerable to practitioners making false claims about their ability to treat or cure serious medical conditions. RH patients may spend considerable time and money on energy healing sessions that offer no real benefit and could delay proper treatment.

The Placebo Effect in Energy Healing

A key factor behind the perceived benefits of energy healing is the placebo effect. The placebo effect occurs when patients experience symptom relief simply because they believe they are receiving treatment, even if the treatment itself has no therapeutic value. The human mind is powerful, and belief in a treatment can lead to real changes in how a patient feels, even if no real medical intervention has occurred.

Energy healing practices, such as Reiki, often create a soothing, calm environment, which can help patients feel more relaxed and less anxious. The act of participating in a ritualized healing process, combined with the care and attention provided by the practitioner, can make patients feel temporarily better. However, this improvement is not due to any manipulation of life energy—it is the result of psychological factors and the brain's response to perceived care.

For RH patients, the placebo effect may lead to short-term relief of symptoms such as anxiety or stress, which can exacerbate hypoglycemic episodes. However, it will not address the underlying metabolic issues causing their condition. Relying on placebo-driven relief rather than evidence-based medical care can result in the worsening of RH symptoms over time, leaving the patient more vulnerable to dangerous blood sugar drops.

Energy Healing and the "Healing" Industry

Energy healing has become part of the larger alternative health industry, which markets treatments as "natural" alternatives to conventional medicine. This industry appeals to individuals who feel disillusioned by mainstream medicine or who are seeking solutions for chronic conditions that are difficult to manage, such as RH.

For patients with RH, the allure of a simple, non-invasive solution to their complex condition can be especially strong. Practitioners of Reiki and similar energy healing methods may take advantage of this vulnerability by promising to relieve symptoms without the need for dietary management or medical interventions. However, these promises are unsubstantiated and not supported by scientific evidence.

Patients with RH should approach any treatment that claims to offer significant relief or a cure with skepticism, especially if the treatment is not backed by clinical research. While energy healing may seem harmless, the financial and emotional costs can be high, and the focus on unproven therapies can distract patients from seeking legitimate medical care.

Conclusion

Energy healing practices like Reiki, which claim to manipulate a person's life energy to alleviate symptoms, are based on pseudoscience. These therapies lack any grounding in biological or medical research, making them ineffective for treating serious metabolic disorders like Reactive Hypoglycemia. While energy healing may provide short-term psychological relief through the placebo effect, it does not address the underlying causes of RH and can delay proper medical care.

RH patients need evidence-based treatments and dietary strategies to manage their condition effectively. Energy healing, with its unproven claims and lack of scientific support, is not a suitable alternative. For those dealing with RH, it is essential to rely on medical advice and scientifically backed treatments rather than being swayed by the false promises of energy healing.

9 Detoxing the Myths

In recent years, detox and cleansing therapies have surged in popularity within alternative medicine circles. These therapies claim to alleviate or even cure various conditions, including digestive disorders, autoimmune issues, and metabolic conditions like Reactive Hypoglycemia (RH). Whether it's liver cleanses, colon cleanses, juice fasts, or special detox diets, these approaches are advertised as magical solutions for a host of ailments. However, for individuals managing chronic conditions like RH, these detox methods not only provide false hope but are also based on pseudoscientific principles that can be dangerous. This chapter explores the myths surrounding detox and cleansing therapies, explains why they are hazardous for individuals with RH, and discusses how the placebo effect often fuels perceived benefits.

The Myth of Detoxification

Detox and cleansing therapies operate on the premise that the body accumulates harmful toxins over time, causing illness and requiring elimination through detox regimens. Proponents of detox diets claim that toxins come from various sources, such as pollution, processed foods, alcohol, heavy metals, medications, and even stress. By undergoing a detox, patients are promised that these toxins will be purged, restoring health and balance.

The problem with this premise is that there is no scientific basis to suggest that the body harbors a significant accumulation of toxins that need to be flushed out. The human body is exceptionally efficient at detoxifying itself through natural processes. The liver, kidneys, lungs, skin, and gastrointestinal tract all work together to process and eliminate waste and toxins daily. The liver metabolizes harmful substances into less toxic forms, the kidneys filter blood and excrete waste through urine, the lungs expel carbon dioxide, and the skin eliminates waste through sweat.

In short, the body already has a highly effective detoxification system. Detox diets or cleanses cannot enhance this process. Claims that juice fasts, colon cleanses, or herbal supplements can rid the body of toxins are misleading and not scientifically substantiated. For individuals with RH, detox diets can lead to serious health risks, exacerbating blood sugar fluctuations and interfering with necessary metabolic functions.

Why Detox Therapies Are Dangerous for RH Patients

Reactive Hypoglycemia involves a sudden drop in blood sugar levels after eating, caused by an abnormal insulin response. Managing RH requires careful dietary planning, regular blood sugar monitoring, and sometimes medication. Detox and cleansing therapies not only fail to address the root causes of RH, but they can also aggravate the condition.

Many detox diets promote extreme calorie restriction, juice fasting, or consuming only specific "cleansing" foods for days or even weeks. These practices deprive the body of essential nutrients, weaken the immune system, and can lead to physical exhaustion. For RH patients, who already deal with fluctuations in energy, fatigue, dizziness, and blood sugar drops, these diets can worsen symptoms and lead to dangerous hypoglycemic episodes.

Dehydration, electrolyte imbalances, and nutrient deficiencies are common side effects of detox diets. For RH patients, these effects can increase the risk of hypoglycemic episodes, leading to confusion, headaches, shakiness, and fainting.

Detox diets that recommend fasting or restricting essential nutrients such as protein and fat can leave RH patients vulnerable to sudden and severe blood sugar crashes.

Some detox regimens also promote herbal supplements that claim to stimulate the liver or colon. Many of these supplements contain laxatives or diuretics, which can lead to diarrhea, dehydration, and worsened fatigue. For RH patients, this can be especially dangerous, as any imbalance in hydration or electrolyte levels can exacerbate blood sugar control problems, increasing the risk of serious complications.

Colon Cleansing: A Particularly Hazardous Trend

Colon cleansing is a particularly dangerous detox trend. Advocates of this practice claim that toxins accumulate in the colon and must be flushed out to restore health. This idea, known as "autointoxication," is based on the outdated theory that waste material in the colon can be reabsorbed into the bloodstream, leading to health problems. Colon cleansing often involves enemas, colonic irrigation, or herbal laxatives to "flush out" these supposed toxins.

There is no scientific evidence to support the need for colon cleansing. The body naturally eliminates waste through bowel movements, and there is no need for intervention unless advised by a healthcare provider for medical reasons, such as before a colonoscopy. Colon cleansing carries significant risks, including dehydration, electrolyte imbalances, infections, and even bowel perforation. These risks can be life-threatening, particularly for RH patients, who already face challenges maintaining metabolic balance.

Additionally, introducing harsh laxatives or undergoing colonic irrigation can disrupt normal gastrointestinal function, leading to further complications in individuals with sensitive digestive systems. For RH patients, maintaining steady and regular nutrient intake is essential to prevent dangerous drops in blood sugar, and disrupting this process through colon cleansing could lead to severe health risks.

Juice Fasting: Nutrient Deficiency and Fatigue

Juice fasting is another common detox method promoted as a way to "cleanse" the body of toxins. Juice fasts typically involve consuming only fruit and vegetable juices for several days or weeks. Advocates claim that this gives the digestive system a break, allowing the body to focus on healing. While fruits and vegetables are packed with nutrients, juice fasts deprive the body of important macronutrients like protein and fat, which are necessary for energy and maintaining muscle mass.

For RH patients, juice fasting can lead to even greater fatigue, muscle weakness, and cognitive impairment. Without adequate protein, fat, and fiber, blood sugar levels can swing dramatically, increasing the risk of hypoglycemic episodes. The high sugar content in fruit juices can cause rapid spikes and crashes in blood sugar levels, which can exacerbate headaches, dizziness, and irritability—symptoms that overlap with RH. Prolonged juice fasting can also lead to dangerous nutrient deficiencies that further worsen metabolic health.

Why People Believe in Detox Therapies

Despite the lack of scientific evidence, detox therapies remain popular for several reasons. The simplicity of the detox narrative—the idea that toxins cause illness and can be easily removed through a cleanse—is appealing to people who are seeking quick solutions. For RH patients, who often face frustrating and slow progress in managing their condition, the promise of a detox as a cure-all is especially enticing.

Testimonials from individuals who claim to feel better after a cleanse play a significant role in perpetuating the belief in detox therapies. However, these testimonials often reflect the placebo effect, temporary dietary changes (such as cutting out processed foods), or the body's natural recovery after short-term fasting or rest. The placebo effect, in particular, is powerful and can lead individuals to believe a treatment is working even when there is no real physical benefit.

Additionally, the wellness industry heavily markets detox

products using fear-based messaging, warning people about the dangers of toxins and emphasizing the need for regular detoxification. This fear, combined with the promise of quick results, drives individuals to try detox regimens, despite the lack of evidence supporting their effectiveness.

The Placebo Effect and Perceived Benefits

The placebo effect plays a significant role in why people feel better after undergoing detox therapies. The act of engaging in a health-promoting ritual, whether it's drinking juice or taking detox supplements, can create a psychological sense of well-being. This perceived improvement in symptoms is often attributed to the detox itself, even though the body's natural recovery or lifestyle changes are likely responsible.

While the placebo effect can lead to short-term psychological relief, it poses risks for RH patients who rely on detox therapies to manage serious metabolic issues. Relying on the placebo effect can delay proper medical treatment and leave symptoms unmanaged, leading to worsened blood sugar control and more frequent hypoglycemic episodes.

Conclusion: Detoxing from Detox Myths

Detox and cleansing therapies are built on pseudoscientific claims that mislead patients into believing that toxins are responsible for their health problems. For individuals with complex metabolic conditions like Reactive Hypoglycemia, these therapies offer false hope and can be dangerous. RH requires careful dietary and medical management, and no detox diet, cleanse, or supplement can regulate insulin responses or stabilize blood sugar levels. By focusing on scientifically backed treatments and rejecting the myths of detox therapies, RH patients can take control of their condition in a safe and effective way.

10 Misleading Nature's Potential

Herbal remedies have long been used in traditional medicine, with many plants and herbs touted for their healing properties. While some herbs are well-documented for providing relief from certain ailments, such as ginger for nausea or echinacea for immune support, using herbal remedies to treat complex metabolic conditions like Reactive Hypoglycemia (RH) veers into dangerous territory. While herbal medicine may seem like a safe, "natural" option, the reality is that not all herbs are beneficial for conditions like RH, and claims that they can treat or cure RH are often unsubstantiated and sometimes harmful.

The Appeal of Herbal Remedies for Chronic Conditions

Herbal medicine appeals to many patients because it offers an alternative to pharmaceuticals, which can come with side effects or be perceived as too invasive. For those with RH, the promise of herbal remedies can seem like a natural and simple solution, especially when managing RH requires strict dietary planning and frequent blood sugar monitoring. Herbal remedies are also marketed as "natural," which appeals to patients who may feel overwhelmed by their condition and seek non-pharmaceutical interventions.

The idea that healing can come from nature resonates deeply with people who are looking for an accessible and non-invasive way to manage chronic health issues. However, it's important to recognize that "natural" does not always mean "safe" or "effective." Many herbal remedies are marketed without sufficient evidence to back their claims, especially when it comes to conditions as complex as RH.

Misleading Claims of Herbal Cures for RH

Despite the lack of scientific evidence, herbal remedies are often marketed as treatments for RH, especially through unregulated online platforms or alternative health practitioners. These claims usually focus on herbs that supposedly balance blood sugar, reduce inflammation, or support metabolic health. Unfortunately, there is no strong clinical evidence to suggest that any herb can "cure" or significantly alleviate RH symptoms.

RH is a metabolic condition caused by an abnormal insulin response that leads to drops in blood sugar after meals. Herbal remedies cannot address the underlying physiological issue of insulin dysregulation, and any claims that herbs can balance blood sugar or stabilize insulin response are unproven. Herbal remedies might have a role in general health maintenance, but they do not have the capacity to treat the underlying causes of RH.

Popular Herbs Promoted for RH

Several herbs are commonly recommended for managing blood sugar and are often falsely promoted as treatments for RH. Here are a few herbs frequently associated with managing blood sugar:

1. **Cinnamon**: This spice is often touted for its potential to lower blood sugar levels. While some studies have shown that cinnamon may help with blood sugar control in type 2 diabetes, its effects on RH are unproven. Moreover, excessive cinnamon consumption can be harmful, leading to liver damage due to its high coumarin content.

2. **Fenugreek**: Fenugreek seeds are promoted as a way to improve insulin sensitivity and lower blood sugar levels. While fenugreek may have some effects on blood sugar,

there is no clear evidence that it can manage the sharp insulin spikes that characterize RH.

3. **Bitter Melon**: Bitter melon is often used in traditional medicine to lower blood sugar, and some small studies suggest it may have a mild effect in managing diabetes. However, it is not a suitable treatment for RH, and its use can lead to gastrointestinal side effects, such as diarrhea or upset stomach.

4. **Gymnema Sylvestre**: This herb is promoted for its ability to lower blood sugar and reduce sugar cravings. While it may help reduce sugar absorption, it does not address the insulin-related causes of RH.

5. **Berberine**: A compound found in certain plants, berberine is often recommended as a natural blood sugar stabilizer. Some studies suggest that it can help lower blood glucose, but there is no research supporting its use in managing RH specifically.

The Danger of Interactions and Side Effects

One of the biggest risks of using herbal remedies to manage RH is the potential for dangerous drug interactions and side effects. Many RH patients may already be taking medications or supplements to manage blood sugar or other symptoms. Introducing herbal remedies without medical supervision can lead to unintended consequences.

For example:

- **St. John's Wort**: Often used for depression, this herb can interfere with the metabolism of many medications, including those used to control blood sugar.

- **Ginkgo Biloba**: While sometimes marketed as a way to improve circulation and brain function, Ginkgo Biloba can increase the risk of bleeding, especially for patients on blood thinners or anticoagulants.

- **Bitter Melon**: While it may lower blood sugar, it can also lead to dangerously low blood sugar levels (hypoglycemia) when combined with other blood sugar-lowering medications or herbs.

Additionally, the unregulated nature of herbal supplements adds to the risk. Unlike pharmaceuticals, herbal remedies are not subjected to rigorous testing for safety, efficacy, or purity. As a result, patients may unknowingly take supplements that are mislabeled, contaminated, or inconsistent in dosage, further complicating their health management.

The Placebo Effect

Many patients who turn to herbal remedies may feel temporary relief, which is often attributed to the placebo effect. The placebo effect occurs when a patient experiences real or perceived improvements in their symptoms simply because they believe the treatment will help. For RH patients, whose symptoms like dizziness, fatigue, or headaches can fluctuate, it is easy to mistake natural symptom improvement for the effects of an herbal remedy.

The placebo effect can provide a sense of relief, but it does not address the root cause of RH. While feeling better psychologically is important, RH patients must recognize that relying on placebo-driven herbal treatments can delay proper medical care, potentially worsening their condition over time.

The Risks of Delaying Effective Treatment

One of the most dangerous aspects of using herbal remedies for RH is the potential delay in receiving effective treatment. Relying solely on herbs may give patients a false sense of security, leading them to postpone necessary dietary changes, medical management, or other proven treatments. While it's natural to seek alternatives, RH requires careful monitoring and management, and relying on herbal supplements can have serious consequences.

When RH is left unmanaged or improperly treated, patients may experience more frequent and severe hypoglycemic episodes, increasing the risk of complications like fainting, confusion, or seizures. Furthermore, chronic episodes of low blood sugar can strain the body and lead to long-term health issues, including cardiovascular problems.

The Herbal Industry and Lack of Regulation

The widespread availability of herbal remedies and the lack of regulation in the supplement industry allow for unchecked marketing of these products. In the United States, for example, the FDA does not regulate herbal supplements to the same extent as prescription medications. This lack of oversight means manufacturers can make broad, unverified claims about their products' benefits without scientific evidence to support them.

Many websites or alternative health practitioners promoting herbal remedies rely heavily on patient testimonials rather than clinical research. While personal stories can be compelling, they do not substitute for controlled, peer-reviewed studies that verify the safety and efficacy of a treatment.

Herbal Medicine: When It Works, When It Doesn't

To be clear, herbal remedies do have their place in medicine. Many modern pharmaceuticals are derived from plants, and certain herbs have been proven effective for specific conditions. For example, peppermint oil is effective for irritable bowel syndrome, and ginger is excellent for nausea relief. However, the distinction lies in the evidence: these herbs have been rigorously studied and have specific, targeted uses.

The problem arises when herbal remedies are promoted as cures for complex metabolic conditions like RH. While some herbs may support general health, they cannot cure or manage the root causes of RH, which involves abnormal insulin response. Herbal remedies may play a complementary role in promoting overall well-being, but they should never replace proven, evidence-based treatments for conditions like RH.

Conclusion: Navigating the Herbal Remedy Landscape

Herbal remedies can offer benefits for general wellness,

but they are not cures for complex conditions like Reactive Hypoglycemia. Patients should exercise caution when considering herbal supplements and always consult with healthcare providers before introducing new herbs into their regimen. Ultimately, a balanced approach that combines evidence-based medicine with informed, safe use of natural remedies is the best way to manage RH effectively.

11 Uncredible Aromatherapy

The use of essential oils has gained widespread popularity in recent years, with claims that these fragrant plant extracts can treat a variety of health problems. From headaches to anxiety, essential oils are marketed as gentle, natural solutions to many ailments. This appeal extends to those with chronic conditions like Reactive Hypoglycemia (RH), a disorder characterized by low blood sugar levels after eating, leading to symptoms such as fatigue, dizziness, headaches, and irritability. Essential oils, such as peppermint or lavender, are often promoted as a means to alleviate these symptoms. However, while essential oils may provide some mild, temporary relief from stress, there is no scientific evidence to support their use as a treatment for the physiological imbalances that cause RH.

In this chapter, we will explore the rise of essential oils as alternative health treatments, examine the pseudoscientific claims surrounding their use for RH, and analyze the risks associated with relying on them for serious metabolic conditions. Although essential oils may have a role in promoting relaxation and reducing mild stress, promoting them as a treatment for RH represents a dangerous form of quackery.

The Popularity of Essential Oils

Essential oils have been used in various cultures for

centuries, primarily for their fragrance, cosmetic uses, and supposed therapeutic properties. Recently, their use has skyrocketed, thanks in part to the global wellness movement. Promoted by multi-level marketing companies and social media influencers, essential oils are now found in homes, health stores, and even mainstream retail chains. The global essential oil market has grown exponentially, fueled by claims that these oils can boost immunity, relieve stress, improve sleep, and even treat chronic illnesses like RH.

For individuals living with the unpredictable nature of RH, the allure of a natural remedy is understandable. Managing low blood sugar can be stressful, and the promise of relief through something as simple as an essential oil is appealing. Essential oils are often associated with calming, soothing properties, which can seem like a harmless and gentle option. While these oils may help with general relaxation or stress reduction, they do not address the root cause of RH, which lies in abnormal insulin response and blood sugar regulation.

Claims of Essential Oils for Reactive Hypoglycemia

Essential oils are often marketed with bold claims, particularly when it comes to managing symptoms related to RH. Oils such as peppermint, lavender, eucalyptus, and frankincense are touted as remedies for headaches, fatigue, dizziness, and anxiety—symptoms commonly experienced by those with RH. For example, peppermint oil is often promoted as a remedy for headaches, with claims that applying it to the temples can reduce pain. Lavender is recommended for anxiety and sleep issues, both of which can be exacerbated by the erratic blood sugar swings seen in RH.

While these oils may help create a calming atmosphere and assist with stress relief, the idea that essential oils can regulate blood sugar or prevent hypoglycemic episodes is entirely unsupported by scientific evidence. Essential oils cannot alter the body's insulin response, improve glucose tolerance, or stabilize blood sugar levels—key elements in managing RH.

The Pseudoscientific Foundation of Essential Oil Claims

The claims made about essential oils for RH are grounded in pseudoscience. Advocates often rely on the appeal to nature fallacy—the belief that because something is natural, it must be effective. This is common in alternative medicine, where anything derived from plants is often seen as inherently beneficial, regardless of scientific support.

However, this belief ignores the complexities of metabolic conditions like RH. RH is caused by an abnormal insulin response that leads to dips in blood sugar levels after meals. Essential oils, no matter how pleasant or relaxing, cannot regulate insulin or stabilize blood glucose levels. The suggestion that simply inhaling or applying an essential oil can treat the physiological issues at the heart of RH lacks any basis in biology or medicine.

Testimonials Versus Actual Outcomes

One reason essential oils have gained popularity is the abundance of testimonials from individuals who claim to have experienced relief. These stories, shared across social media, blogs, and essential oil marketing platforms, often describe how oils helped manage headaches, reduced fatigue, or eased stress. These testimonials can be incredibly persuasive, particularly for people who are searching for non-pharmaceutical solutions to RH symptoms.

However, it's important to differentiate between anecdotal evidence and scientific proof. Testimonials are not the same as research-backed evidence. They are often subject to the placebo effect—where a person feels better simply because they expect the treatment to work. For instance, inhaling a calming scent like lavender may provide a temporary sense of relaxation, which could reduce the perception of fatigue or stress associated with RH. This, however, does not mean that the essential oil is treating the underlying cause of RH.

Essential oil companies often leverage these testimonials as marketing tools, creating a cycle where more people try the oils based on personal stories rather than scientific evidence. This becomes particularly dangerous for individuals with serious health conditions like RH, who may delay seeking effective medical treatments in favor of unproven remedies.

The Risks of Essential Oils for RH Patients

While essential oils are generally considered safe when used properly, they are not without risks—particularly for individuals with chronic conditions like RH. One of the primary concerns is that essential oils offer no real treatment for the underlying cause of RH, which is the abnormal insulin response leading to drops in blood sugar. Focusing on essential oils rather than proven dietary or medical interventions can result in delayed or inadequate management of RH, worsening symptoms, and increasing the risk of severe hypoglycemic episodes.

Additionally, essential oils can cause allergic reactions, skin irritations, or respiratory issues, particularly when used improperly. For instance, peppermint oil applied directly to the skin without dilution can cause irritation or burns, while inhaling large amounts of certain oils, such as eucalyptus, can lead to respiratory distress in sensitive individuals. Ingesting essential oils, which is sometimes recommended by alternative health advocates, can be especially dangerous, as high concentrations of essential oils can be toxic and damage internal organs.

Furthermore, the financial cost of essential oils can be a burden, especially when marketed as ongoing treatments for chronic conditions like RH. Essential oils are often sold at high prices through multi-level marketing companies, which can lead vulnerable individuals to spend significant sums of money on products that provide no actual health benefits.

The Placebo Effect and Perceived Benefits

The placebo effect plays a significant role in the perceived benefits of essential oils, particularly for conditions like RH. The placebo effect occurs when a person experiences a perceived improvement in their condition simply because they believe the treatment is working, even if the treatment has no physiological impact. For RH patients, the placebo effect may lead to temporary relief of stress or anxiety, which are common symptoms associated with blood sugar fluctuations.

The calming nature of using essential oils, combined with the pleasant sensory experience of smelling fragrances or engaging in self-care rituals, can enhance the placebo effect. However, this temporary psychological relief does not address the physiological causes of RH, such as insulin dysregulation. Mistaking the placebo effect for real improvement can prevent patients from seeking the medical or dietary interventions necessary to properly manage RH.

Conclusion: Essential Oils Offer False Hope for RH

While essential oils may provide temporary relaxation and stress relief, they are not a treatment for Reactive Hypoglycemia. The claims made by essential oil companies and alternative health advocates are not supported by scientific evidence, and relying on these products for RH management can delay necessary care. For individuals with RH, it is crucial to rely on evidence-based medicine and proper dietary management to regulate blood sugar levels and reduce hypoglycemic episodes.

Essential oils can have a place in personal wellness routines, but they should not be viewed as a cure or treatment for serious metabolic conditions like RH. As with any medical condition, patients should consult with healthcare professionals to ensure they are following safe and effective treatments that address the root cause of their symptoms.

12 Needles and Nonsense

Acupuncture, an ancient practice rooted in traditional Chinese medicine (TCM), has gained popularity as an alternative therapy for a wide range of conditions, from chronic pain to anxiety. Proponents claim that acupuncture, which involves inserting thin needles into specific points on the body, can alleviate a variety of health problems. More recently, acupuncture has been promoted as a treatment for metabolic disorders, including Reactive Hypoglycemia (RH). Supporters argue that it can help manage symptoms such as dizziness, headaches, and fatigue—common issues for those with RH. However, despite its long history and growing popularity, there is little scientific evidence to support acupuncture's efficacy in treating serious metabolic conditions like RH.

This chapter will explore the origins of acupuncture, the claims made about its effectiveness for RH, and the dangers of relying on acupuncture as a treatment. We will also examine the pseudoscientific foundation of acupuncture, the role of the placebo effect, and the risks associated with delaying proper medical care in favor of this alternative therapy.

The Origins and Practice of Acupuncture

Acupuncture has its roots in traditional Chinese medicine, a system of healing that dates back thousands of years. According to TCM, the body has a vital life force called "qi" (pronounced "chee") that flows through pathways known as meridians. When the flow of qi is blocked or imbalanced, illness is believed to occur. Acupuncturists claim that by inserting needles into specific points along these meridians, they can restore balance to qi, promoting healing and alleviating symptoms.

In modern times, acupuncture has expanded beyond its TCM origins and is widely practiced in Western countries. It is frequently promoted as a treatment for pain management, stress relief, and various other conditions. In some cases, acupuncture is used as a complementary therapy alongside conventional treatments, but in other instances, it is marketed as a stand-alone solution for complex medical conditions.

For those living with Reactive Hypoglycemia, acupuncture may seem appealing due to its non-invasive nature and the promise of natural healing. However, while acupuncture may offer some relief for pain or stress, it is not a proven treatment for the metabolic imbalances that underlie RH.

Claims About Acupuncture for Reactive Hypoglycemia

Proponents of acupuncture often claim that the practice can alleviate symptoms associated with RH, including headaches, fatigue, and dizziness. These symptoms are common among RH patients and can be difficult to manage through conventional methods alone, particularly when dietary interventions fall short. As a result, some RH patients may turn to acupuncture, hoping it will provide an alternative form of symptom management.

Acupuncturists often argue that acupuncture can "release" pain, reduce inflammation, and improve energy levels by restoring the flow of qi. Specific acupuncture points on the stomach, liver, and spleen are frequently targeted in treatments for RH patients, as these are believed to play a role in digestion and metabolism according to TCM principles. Some practitioners also claim that acupuncture can regulate blood sugar levels, a key factor in managing RH.

These claims, however, lack scientific support. While some patients may experience temporary relief from acupuncture, there is no credible evidence to suggest that it can address the root cause of RH, which is an abnormal insulin response to carbohydrate intake. Acupuncture cannot alter the body's metabolic processes or regulate glucose levels, making it an ineffective treatment for RH.

The Pseudoscientific Foundation of Acupuncture

Acupuncture is based on concepts that have no grounding in modern scientific understanding of the human body. The notion of qi and meridians, for example, has never been observed or demonstrated in any scientific study. Despite its long history, there is no anatomical or physiological evidence to support the existence of qi or that it flows through the body in specific pathways.

Some modern acupuncturists have attempted to explain acupuncture's effects in more scientific terms, suggesting that the insertion of needles may stimulate the nervous system, release endorphins (natural painkillers), or improve blood circulation. However, these explanations are speculative and do not account for how acupuncture would directly affect the metabolic imbalances that cause RH.

Moreover, clinical trials on acupuncture have generally found that its effects are no better than placebo. In studies where participants received "sham" acupuncture—where needles are inserted randomly or superficially—patients reported similar levels of symptom relief as those who received real acupuncture. This suggests that the benefits of acupuncture are largely attributable to the placebo effect, rather than any specific therapeutic action.

The Placebo Effect and Acupuncture

The placebo effect is a well-documented phenomenon where patients experience real improvements in their symptoms after receiving a treatment with no therapeutic value. The power of the placebo effect lies in the patient's belief that the treatment will work. In the case of acupuncture, the ritual of needle insertion, the calm environment, and the practitioner's reassurance can lead to a strong placebo response.

For patients with RH, the placebo effect can offer temporary relief from stress, anxiety, or even mild fatigue. This is especially true for symptoms like headaches, which can be exacerbated by stress or tension. However, the placebo effect does not address the root cause of RH, which involves abnormal insulin response and blood sugar regulation.

The danger of relying on acupuncture for RH is that it may give patients false hope. While they may feel better in the short term, their condition is not being treated, and their symptoms could worsen over time. The temporary relief provided by acupuncture may also lead some patients to delay seeking appropriate medical care, which could result in more serious health issues down the road.

Risks of Acupuncture for RH Patients

While acupuncture is generally considered safe when performed by trained practitioners, it is not without risks—especially for individuals with underlying metabolic disorders like RH. One of the primary risks associated with acupuncture is that it may provide a false sense of security, causing patients to delay or avoid evidence-based treatments.

RH is a condition that requires careful dietary management and, in some cases, medical intervention to stabilize blood sugar levels. If patients rely on acupuncture instead of following proven medical advice or nutritional guidelines, they may experience more frequent and severe hypoglycemic episodes. Delaying proper care can lead to serious consequences, including fainting, seizures, or even coma.

Additionally, there are minor physical risks associated with acupuncture, such as infection or bruising, particularly if needles are not properly sterilized. While these risks are rare, they are still a concern, especially for individuals with compromised immune systems or other underlying health conditions.

Testimonials Versus Scientific Evidence

As with many alternative therapies, acupuncture is often promoted through personal testimonials rather than scientific evidence. Patients who report feeling better after acupuncture treatments may attribute their improvement to the needles, when in fact their symptoms may have improved on their own or as a result of the placebo effect. Testimonials can be persuasive, particularly when they come from individuals who share similar struggles.

However, it is important to recognize the limitations of anecdotal evidence. Just because one person reports feeling better after acupuncture does not mean that the treatment is effective for everyone, or that it addresses the underlying cause of their condition. RH is a complex metabolic disorder that requires medical intervention, and there is no credible evidence to suggest that acupuncture can regulate blood sugar or improve insulin sensitivity.

The Dangers of False Hope

One of the most concerning aspects of acupuncture for RH is the false hope it offers to patients. RH can cause debilitating symptoms and, in some cases, serious complications if not properly managed. Patients who are desperate for relief may turn to acupuncture in the hopes of finding an alternative solution to their condition.

Unfortunately, acupuncture does not offer a cure for RH. While it may provide temporary relief from some symptoms, it cannot address the metabolic imbalances that cause hypoglycemia. Relying on acupuncture as a treatment can prevent patients from seeking the medical care they need, potentially leading to worse outcomes.

For patients with RH, it is essential to pursue evidence-based treatments that have been proven to be effective in managing the condition. This includes proper dietary management, regular blood sugar monitoring, and, in some cases, medication. While acupuncture may have a place in complementary care for managing stress or mild discomfort, it should not be viewed as a substitute for medical treatment.

Conclusion: Acupuncture and the Illusion of Healing

Acupuncture may offer a temporary reprieve from certain symptoms, but it does not provide a solution for Reactive Hypoglycemia. The practice is based on principles that lack scientific support, and its effects are largely attributable to the placebo effect. While acupuncture is generally safe, it carries risks for patients with serious health conditions, and its promotion as a treatment for RH represents a dangerous form of quackery.

For RH patients, the most important step is to seek evidence-based treatments that address the underlying cause of their condition. While alternative therapies like acupuncture may offer short-term relief, they cannot replace the medical interventions necessary to manage RH symptoms effectively. By focusing on proven treatments and working with qualified healthcare providers, patients can ensure they are receiving the best possible care for their condition.

13 A Breath of False Hope

Ozone therapy has gained popularity as an alternative treatment that promises to cure or alleviate a range of conditions, from chronic pain to infections and even metabolic disorders like Reactive Hypoglycemia (RH). Proponents claim that ozone therapy can increase oxygen levels in the body, boost the immune system, and improve overall health by addressing the root causes of illness. However, much like other alternative treatments, ozone therapy is not backed by credible scientific evidence and, in some cases, it poses significant health risks. In this chapter, we will explore the rise of ozone therapy, examine the claims made by its advocates, and discuss the dangers it presents, especially for individuals with conditions like Reactive Hypoglycemia.

The Origins and Concept of Ozone Therapy

Ozone (O_3) is a molecule composed of three oxygen atoms. While oxygen (O_2) is essential for life, ozone is a toxic gas when inhaled in large quantities, as it is highly reactive and can cause damage to the respiratory system. Despite its toxic nature, ozone has been used for industrial purposes such as water purification and sterilization, due to its ability to kill bacteria and viruses. This industrial application has led some alternative health practitioners to believe that ozone could have medical benefits for humans, under the assumption that what kills harmful microorganisms could also heal the body.

Ozone therapy involves introducing ozone into the body through various methods, including insufflation (blowing ozone into body cavities), injections, or autohemotherapy (mixing a patient's blood with ozone and re-injecting it). Practitioners claim that ozone therapy can increase the oxygen content in the blood, enhancing the body's ability to heal itself by boosting circulation, improving immune function, and reducing inflammation.

For patients with Reactive Hypoglycemia, ozone therapy is sometimes marketed as a way to stabilize blood sugar levels, reduce inflammation, and support overall metabolic health. Proponents argue that by increasing oxygen in the blood, ozone therapy can help the body manage glucose levels more effectively, thus reducing episodes of hypoglycemia. However, these claims lack any credible scientific basis and ignore the complex nature of Reactive Hypoglycemia, which involves abnormal insulin responses to food intake.

Dubious Claims: Ozone Therapy for Reactive Hypoglycemia

Ozone therapy is marketed as a treatment for numerous conditions, including autoimmune diseases, infections, chronic pain, and metabolic disorders like RH. Practitioners suggest that increasing the amount of oxygen in the bloodstream can help improve metabolic function and reduce hypoglycemic episodes by supporting better glucose regulation. Some even claim that ozone therapy can reduce oxidative stress in the body and repair damage to insulin-producing cells.

However, these claims are not supported by any credible scientific evidence. Reactive Hypoglycemia is a condition where the body produces too much insulin in response to carbohydrate consumption, causing blood sugar levels to drop too quickly. The idea that increasing oxygen in the bloodstream through ozone therapy could influence insulin response or stabilize glucose levels has no scientific foundation. Ozone therapy cannot change the body's underlying insulin regulation, which is the core issue in RH.

Moreover, ozone therapy has not been shown to have any impact on the metabolic processes involved in blood sugar regulation. While oxygen is vital for cellular function, increasing the amount of oxygen in the blood through ozone therapy does not translate into better control of insulin or blood sugar. Claims that ozone therapy can repair damaged tissues or enhance glucose metabolism are misleading at best and dangerous at worst.

The Dangers of Ozone Therapy

Ozone therapy is not only ineffective for treating conditions like Reactive Hypoglycemia; it is also potentially harmful. Ozone is a highly reactive molecule, and when introduced into the body, it can lead to oxidative stress, which occurs when there are too many free radicals (unstable molecules that can damage cells) and not enough antioxidants to neutralize them. This oxidative damage can harm proteins, DNA, and other cellular structures, leading to inflammation and the breakdown of healthy tissues.

For patients with Reactive Hypoglycemia, whose metabolic systems are already compromised, the introduction of ozone could exacerbate oxidative stress and inflammation, potentially worsening symptoms. Oxidative stress has been linked to a variety of chronic conditions, including diabetes and metabolic disorders, so using a treatment that increases oxidative damage is counterproductive for individuals with RH.

In addition to oxidative stress, there are other risks associated with ozone therapy. Ozone therapy can cause inflammation, tissue damage, and even life-threatening complications when injected or introduced into body cavities. The inhalation of ozone, even in small amounts, can irritate the respiratory system, leading to coughing, shortness of breath, and lung damage. For individuals with underlying health conditions, these risks are heightened.

Another significant danger of ozone therapy is the risk of

infection, especially when the therapy involves injections or autohemotherapy (drawing blood, mixing it with ozone, and reinjecting it). Anytime the skin is pierced or blood is handled outside of the body, there is a risk of introducing harmful bacteria or viruses into the bloodstream. If proper sterilization procedures are not followed, this can lead to serious infections, which could be especially harmful to someone already dealing with a metabolic disorder like RH.

Lack of Scientific Evidence

Despite the bold claims made by advocates of ozone therapy, there is little to no scientific evidence to support its use for any medical condition, let alone for complex metabolic disorders like Reactive Hypoglycemia. While ozone has been studied for its ability to kill bacteria and viruses in environmental and industrial settings, these findings do not translate to human health treatments. There is no credible research demonstrating that ozone therapy can improve oxygen levels in a way that would benefit people with RH, nor is there any evidence that it can cure or manage the condition.

The U.S. Food and Drug Administration (FDA) has explicitly warned against the use of ozone therapy, stating that ozone is a toxic gas with no known useful medical application. The FDA has cautioned that the use of ozone in medical treatments can lead to severe respiratory complications and other health problems. Despite these warnings, ozone therapy continues to be promoted by alternative health practitioners, often at the expense of patients' health and safety.

The Role of the Placebo Effect

As with many alternative therapies, the placebo effect plays a major role in the perceived benefits of ozone therapy. Patients who undergo ozone therapy may report feeling better afterward, but this improvement is often due to the placebo effect rather than any real physiological changes. The placebo effect occurs when a patient's belief in the treatment leads to a perceived improvement in symptoms, even if the treatment itself has no therapeutic value.

For patients with Reactive Hypoglycemia, the placebo effect can offer temporary relief from symptoms like fatigue or anxiety. However, this relief does not address the underlying insulin dysregulation that causes hypoglycemic episodes. Relying on ozone therapy may lead patients to delay more effective treatments, putting them at greater risk for severe hypoglycemic events.

Ethical Concerns Surrounding Ozone Therapy

One of the most troubling aspects of ozone therapy is the ethical implications of promoting a treatment that has no scientific backing and carries significant risks. Patients with RH are often desperate for solutions, particularly if conventional treatments or dietary changes have not fully resolved their symptoms. This desperation can make them vulnerable to alternative health practitioners who offer false hope through unproven therapies like ozone.

Promoting ozone therapy as a cure for Reactive Hypoglycemia is not only misleading but also potentially harmful. Patients who believe in the promises of ozone therapy may forgo or delay seeking legitimate medical treatment, putting their health at risk. Moreover, the financial costs of ozone therapy can be significant, as practitioners often charge high fees for treatments that have no proven benefit.

Conclusion: Ozone Therapy as a False Hope

Ozone therapy is yet another alternative treatment that offers false hope to patients with conditions like Reactive Hypoglycemia. Despite claims that it can increase oxygen levels, reduce inflammation, and improve glucose regulation, there is no credible scientific evidence to support the use of ozone therapy for any medical condition. In fact, ozone therapy carries significant risks, including oxidative stress, infection, and respiratory damage.

For patients with RH, relying on ozone therapy is

particularly dangerous. Reactive Hypoglycemia is a complex metabolic disorder that requires careful dietary management and medical supervision. Pursuing unproven therapies like ozone can delay necessary treatment and put patients at risk for serious health complications. As with any medical treatment, it is essential for patients to seek evidence-based care from qualified healthcare providers, rather than falling prey to pseudoscientific claims and ineffective therapies.

14 How to Research on Your Own

When diagnosed with a complex condition like Reactive Hypoglycemia (RH), finding accurate and reliable information becomes crucial for navigating treatment options and making informed decisions about your health. The internet is filled with a mix of credible scientific resources and misleading pseudoscience. For patients with RH, knowing how to research effectively and avoid misinformation can significantly improve your management of the condition and quality of life.

This chapter will provide essential tools to critically evaluate medical information on RH, navigate peer-reviewed journals, and understand statistics so you can discern which studies are credible. We will also explore how to avoid "quack" journals and pseudoscientific articles disguised as legitimate sources of medical research.

Understanding Peer-Reviewed Journals

The term "peer-reviewed" is often regarded as the gold standard for scientific literature. A peer-reviewed journal means that before a study is published, it is reviewed by other experts in the field to assess its methodology, accuracy, and contribution to the body of research. However, not all journals that claim to be peer-reviewed are reputable, and not all peer-reviewed studies are flawless.

Characteristics of a Legitimate Peer-Reviewed Journal

- **Reputation:** Legitimate peer-reviewed journals are often affiliated with reputable academic institutions or well-known publishers, such as Wiley, Springer, or Elsevier.

- **Impact Factor:** The impact factor measures how often articles in a journal are cited by other researchers. While not perfect, higher impact factors suggest more reputable journals. Journals with an impact factor above 1.0 are considered credible, while prestigious medical journals may have impact factors above 50.

- **Indexed in Databases:** Legitimate journals are often indexed in reputable databases like PubMed, Scopus, or Web of Science. These databases have strict criteria, reducing the likelihood of pseudoscientific or predatory journals being listed.

How to Spot Predatory or Quack Journals

Unfortunately, the rise of the internet has led to an increase in pseudo-journals, or "predatory journals," that masquerade as legitimate scientific sources. These journals may claim to be peer-reviewed but often skip the peer-review process, lack scientific integrity, and are driven by financial gain.

Red Flags for Predatory Journals:

- **Unsolicited Emails:** If you receive emails inviting you to submit papers or review articles for a journal you've never heard of, this is often a sign of a predatory journal.

- **High Fees:** Predatory journals often charge high publication fees without providing proper peer review. While some reputable journals charge for open-access publication, predatory journals exist primarily to collect these fees.

- **Quick Review Process:** Journals that claim to review and publish articles within days or weeks should raise suspicion. Proper peer review takes time to ensure the study's quality.

- **Lack of Transparency:** If you cannot find clear information about a journal's editorial board, affiliations, or peer-review process, it is best to avoid it.

- **Bogus Impact Factors:** Some predatory journals fabricate their impact factors. To verify a journal's true impact factor, check reliable sources like Clarivate's Journal Citation Reports (JCR).

Navigating Statistics and Medical Research

Reading a medical journal article is one thing; understanding the data is another. Many journal articles use complex statistics that can be difficult for non-experts to interpret. Knowing basic statistical terms can help you determine whether a study's findings are credible or misleading.

Key Statistical Terms to Know:

- **P-Value:** The p-value measures the probability that the study's results are due to chance. A p-value of less than 0.05 is often considered statistically significant.

- **Confidence Interval (CI):** This provides a range within which the true result likely falls. A narrow CI suggests more precise results.

- **Sample Size:** Larger sample sizes provide more reliable results, as they reduce the chance of random variations.

- **Relative Risk (RR) and Odds Ratio (OR):** These statistics measure the strength of association between a treatment and an outcome. An RR or OR of 1.0 means no effect, while values higher or lower suggest increased or decreased risk, respectively.

Identifying Reliable Research

Once you understand the basics of peer-reviewed journals and statistical terms, you can begin to critically assess research articles. Here are tips for determining the reliability of a study:

- **Look for Randomized Controlled Trials (RCTs):** These studies, where participants are randomly assigned to treatment or control groups, are the gold standard for clinical research.

- **Check for Meta-Analyses or Systematic Reviews:** These types of studies compile data from multiple studies to provide a broader conclusion, making them more reliable.

- **Assess Author Credentials:** Look for respected researchers in the field of RH or metabolic disorders. Check whether they have a history of publishing in credible journals.

- **Review Funding Sources:** Be cautious if the study was funded by companies with a financial interest in the outcome, such as supplement manufacturers.

Spotting Misleading Research and False Statistics

Not all research is trustworthy. Some studies, particularly those published in predatory journals, may manipulate statistics or selectively report data to make a treatment seem more effective than it is.

Warning Signs of Unreliable Research:

- **Cherry-Picking Data:** Some studies report only favorable results and ignore data that contradicts their hypothesis.

- **Lack of Control Group:** Without a control group, it is impossible to know if a treatment works or if the results are due to other factors.

- **Small Sample Sizes or Short Duration:** Studies with few participants or short follow-ups may not provide meaningful information.

- **Conflicts of Interest:** If a study's authors or funding sources stand to benefit from positive results, take the findings with caution.

Using Quackwatch and Other Resources to Avoid Pseudoscience

Navigating medical research can be overwhelming, especially for those unfamiliar with the field. Quackwatch is a valuable resource for identifying pseudoscientific and fraudulent health claims. Founded by Dr. Stephen Barrett, Quackwatch highlights the lack of evidence behind many popular alternative treatments.

Other reliable resources include:

- **National Institutes of Health (NIH):** Provides extensive, science-based resources on medical conditions and treatments.

- **Cochrane Library:** Publishes systematic reviews of clinical trials, offering high-quality evidence on treatments.

- **PubMed:** A database of biomedical literature, including peer-reviewed journal articles.

Conclusion

Navigating medical research while managing a condition like Reactive Hypoglycemia can be challenging, but by understanding how to evaluate peer-reviewed journals, interpret statistics, and avoid pseudoscience, you can make better-informed decisions. Always critically assess the information you encounter, and rely on reputable resources like PubMed and Quackwatch to ensure your treatment choices are based on solid evidence. By doing so, you can avoid false hope and quackery, ensuring that you receive the most effective care for your condition.

15 Proven Treatments for RH

Reactive Hypoglycemia (RH) is a condition characterized by a drop in blood sugar levels that occurs a few hours after eating. It can be challenging to manage, but with the right treatment approach, individuals can effectively control their symptoms and maintain stable blood sugar levels. While there's no cure for RH, proven treatments focus on diet, lifestyle changes, and sometimes medication. In this chapter, we will outline 12 proven strategies that can help you manage RH effectively.

1. Balanced, Low-Glycemic Diet

The cornerstone of managing RH is adopting a balanced diet that emphasizes low-glycemic foods. Low-glycemic foods digest more slowly, leading to a more gradual rise in blood sugar. These include whole grains, legumes, vegetables, and fruits like berries and apples. Avoid high-glycemic foods such as sugary snacks, white bread, and processed foods that cause blood sugar to spike and crash. Eating complex carbohydrates combined with protein and healthy fats at each meal helps maintain a steady blood glucose level and prevents the rapid drops that cause RH symptoms.

2. Frequent, Smaller Meals

Instead of eating large meals three times a day, RH patients benefit from consuming smaller, frequent meals every 3–4 hours. This approach prevents significant blood sugar fluctuations and helps keep glucose levels stable throughout the day. Meals should include a balance of protein, fiber, and fat, which slows digestion and ensures a steady release of glucose into the bloodstream.

3. Protein-Rich Meals

Adding lean proteins to every meal can help stabilize blood sugar by slowing down the digestion of carbohydrates. Good protein sources include lean meats, fish, eggs, nuts, seeds, and plant-based options like tofu and legumes. Combining protein with complex carbohydrates can reduce the likelihood of experiencing blood sugar crashes after meals.

4. Avoiding Sugary Foods and Drinks

One of the most critical strategies for managing RH is to avoid foods and beverages high in sugar. Sugary foods can cause a rapid spike in blood glucose levels, followed by a sharp drop, leading to hypoglycemia. This includes candies, pastries, sugary drinks, and refined carbohydrates like white bread and pasta. Instead, focus on whole, unprocessed foods that provide a more stable energy source.

5. Fiber-Rich Diet

Eating foods rich in fiber is essential for slowing the absorption of sugars in the digestive tract. High-fiber foods like vegetables, legumes, whole grains, and fruits (such as berries and apples) help prevent rapid rises in blood sugar. Fiber also contributes to a feeling of fullness, which can help regulate appetite and reduce the likelihood of overeating, which can trigger hypoglycemia.

6. Regular Physical Activity

Exercise can help improve insulin sensitivity and regulate blood sugar levels. Moderate exercise, such as walking, cycling, or swimming, is generally beneficial for managing RH. However, it's important not to engage in intense exercise on an empty stomach, as this can exacerbate hypoglycemia. Instead, aim to exercise after eating a balanced meal or snack to help stabilize blood glucose levels.

7. Avoiding High-Carbohydrate Meals

Meals that are high in refined carbohydrates can cause a rapid increase in blood sugar, followed by a sharp drop. To prevent this, RH patients should avoid meals that consist primarily of starchy or sugary foods. Instead, meals should include a combination of protein, fiber, and healthy fats to help slow down the absorption of glucose and keep blood sugar levels steady.

8. Stress Management

Chronic stress can impact blood sugar regulation, as stress hormones like cortisol and adrenaline can cause blood glucose levels to fluctuate. RH patients should focus on stress-reducing activities like deep breathing exercises, meditation, yoga, or even taking a walk. Managing stress is essential for overall health and can help reduce the frequency of hypoglycemic episodes.

9. Hydration and Electrolyte Balance

Dehydration can impair the body's ability to regulate blood sugar. Drinking plenty of water throughout the day is essential for maintaining stable blood sugar levels. In addition to staying hydrated, some RH patients may benefit from maintaining proper electrolyte balance, particularly if they experience symptoms like dizziness or weakness during hypoglycemia. Potassium-rich foods like bananas and avocados, along with magnesium from leafy greens or supplements, may support overall blood sugar stability.

10. Medication for Severe Cases

While dietary changes are typically the first line of treatment for RH, some patients with more severe cases may require medication. For example, drugs like acarbose may be prescribed to slow down the digestion of carbohydrates and prevent post-meal blood sugar spikes. Other medications may target insulin sensitivity or slow gastric emptying. However, medication should only be used under the guidance of a healthcare provider and in combination with dietary and lifestyle changes.

11. Avoiding Alcohol

Alcohol consumption can lower blood sugar levels, particularly when consumed on an empty stomach. For RH patients, alcohol can exacerbate symptoms of hypoglycemia, including dizziness, weakness, and confusion. It is generally recommended that individuals with RH either avoid alcohol entirely or consume it in moderation with food to minimize the risk of a hypoglycemic episode.

12. Continuous Glucose Monitoring (CGM)

Using a continuous glucose monitor (CGM) can be incredibly helpful for RH patients, as it provides real-time data on blood glucose levels throughout the day. A CGM can alert patients when their blood sugar is dropping, allowing them to take action before symptoms of hypoglycemia set in. This technology is particularly beneficial for identifying patterns in blood glucose fluctuations and tailoring diet and lifestyle strategies to better manage RH.

Avoiding Misinformation and Quack Treatments

While these 12 treatments are backed by scientific evidence and clinical practice, RH patients must be cautious of alternative treatments that claim to "cure" the condition without any scientific basis. Unproven treatments can provide false hope and distract from effective management strategies. For example, therapies such as detox diets, herbal remedies, or energy healing have no proven benefit for RH and may lead patients to delay or neglect proper treatment.

By focusing on evidence-based treatments, such as dietary changes, glucose monitoring, and physical activity, RH patients can manage their symptoms and improve their quality of life. Working closely with a healthcare provider is essential for developing an individualized treatment plan that addresses the specific needs of each patient.

In conclusion, managing RH involves a combination of

proven strategies that focus on stabilizing blood sugar levels through diet, lifestyle changes, and, in some cases, medication. By avoiding unproven remedies and relying on evidence-based treatments, patients can take control of their health and effectively manage the challenges of living with reactive hypoglycemia.

16 Conclusion

As we conclude our exploration of Reactive Hypoglycemia and the challenges associated with navigating treatment options, it's essential to understand the landscape of pseudoscience and its potential risks. Patients facing serious conditions like Chiari malformation often encounter promises of "miracle cures" that lack scientific foundation. We hope this book has empowered you with strategies for discerning credible, evidence-based treatments from unsupported claims, ensuring your journey toward wellness remains safe and informed.

Appendix: Tips for How to Avoid Pseudoscience

Living with a serious medical condition, such as Reactive Hypoglycemia, comes with its share of challenges. It is not only physically exhausting but also presents challenges to medical therapy. Unfortunately, this journey becomes even more demanding due to the rise of pseudoscientific "treatments" that promise miraculous cures but often lack scientific evidence. So, how exactly will you differentiate between proven medical treatments and potentially dangerous pseudoscientific claims? Read on to make informed decisions.

Pseudoscience vs. Evidence Based Medicine

Evidence-based medicine lays its foundation on rigorous scientific research, clinical trials, and peer-reviewed studies published in the literature. All these exhaustive steps are taken to ensure the safety of patients.

On the other hand, pseudoscientific therapies are based on mere beliefs and have no profound scientific evidence to support the claims. Even the claims are mostly anecdotal, untested, or even disproven.

Here are some of the most prominent warning signs when making a distinction between a genuine treatment and a pseudoscientific claim.

- **Overly Optimistic Results**

- Treatments claiming to cure serious or impossible-to-cure diseases are red flags.

- **Medical Science Unknown**

- If you can't find any peer-reviewed research or legitimate medical recommendations on the treatment, it is best to be suspicious.

- **Equivocation of Language**

- Terms like "energy healing," "detoxifying the body," or "holistic re-alignment" usually pose a red flag for pseudoscience.

- **Personal Testimonials**

Testimonials are highly persuasive but cannot be considered evidence. These are mostly biased and are not a substitute for scientific research.

Steps to Evaluate a Potential Therapy

Reliable Medical Databases

PubMed and other medical research databases are some of the best ways to confirm whether a treatment is credible or not. The NIH maintains the database, which contains millions of peer-reviewed studies. If a proposed treatment has been evaluated and validated, you will most likely find it on PubMed.

How to use PubMed: Proceed to PubMed.gov and input the treatment combined with your condition. For example, "cranial therapy Reactive Hypoglycemia." Locate any articles that have appeared in peer-reviewed medical journals and determine if there is clinical evidence.

Reputable Health Organizations

Credible health organizations like the Mayo Clinic and the National Institutes of Health can provide information on proven treatments and the risks associated with alternative treatments. The websites update disease, medicine, and alternative treatment databases daily.

Discuss With Your Healthcare Provider

Talk to a primary care physician or specialist before attempting any therapy. Most physicians know alternative therapies and can explain why certain interventions should not be encouraged.

Ask your doctor during your consultation these questions:

- *"What evidence is there to support this treatment?"*

- *"Is there any known danger associated with it?"*

- *Do you support this approach for a patient with my condition?"*

Find Systematic Reviews and Consensus Statements

A systematic review evaluates large amounts of research to judge the effectiveness of treatments. For example, The Cochrane Library is a good resource because it focuses on systematic reviews of the results of large volumes of research that evaluate health interventions.

Be Cautious of the Books That Advocate the "Miracle Cure

Even books or articles claim to "cure" serious conditions based merely on extreme dietary changes or unproven treatments. In general, some types of dietary change can improve quality of life and contribute to wellness; however, they seldom represent a complete cure.

ABOUT THE AUTHORS

Cheryl White has been a dedicated health science writer for more than 30 years. With an undergraduate degree in Health Sciences and two master's degrees, Cheryl's passion for helping people live healthier lives comes through in her writing, making complex health issues understandable and accessible for all readers.

Shane Wilson is a dedicated medical professional with a passion for debunking health myths and pseudoscientific practices. With over three years of experience in crafting well-researched, engaging medical content, Shane aims to empower readers with accurate, evidence-based information. His writing is a compelling blend of expertise and clarity, making complex medical topics accessible to all.

Excerpt from Reactive Hypoglycemia: Your 5 Step Recovery Plan

Allison Francis, MAT & Betty Johnson, MD (Ed.)

Five Steps to Recovery:

1. Get a diagnosis
2. Eliminate these from your diet
3. Keep a journal and monitor your blood sugar
4. Tailor your diet
5. De-stress with complementary and alternative medicine techniques

Step One: Get a diagnosis

Getting a diagnosis of reactive hypoglycemia is the essential first step in the 5-Step Recovery Plan. Knowing the cause of your reactive hypoglycemia is crucial because it helps determine the most effective treatment approach. This chapter will discuss the diagnostic tools available to identify underlying conditions—like insulin sensitivity, prediabetes, or even rare disorders like insulinoma—that may be at play. Each diagnosis can shape your approach to managing symptoms, preventing complications, and improving quality of life.

Overcoming Barriers to Diagnosis

Not everyone has access to a healthcare provider. If seeing a doctor feels out of reach, whether due to cost or lack of insurance, you're not alone. Options for low-cost testing are available through community health clinics, nonprofit organizations, and even telemedicine providers. Many clinics offer sliding-scale fees based on income, and health fairs and free screenings often provide essential tests for free. Understanding these options means you can still make progress, even if traditional healthcare access is limited.

Diagnostic Methods for Reactive Hypoglycemia

Let's dive into the diagnostic methods that can help determine the cause of your reactive hypoglycemia. These methods range from at-home monitoring to specialized medical testing.

1. Hyperglucidic Breakfast Test

The Hyperglucidic Breakfast Test, developed by Dr. Jean-Frédéric Brun, is widely used in Europe as a reliable diagnostic tool. This test replicates a typical high-carb meal that may induce hypoglycemic symptoms. The test involves a meal of bread, butter, jam, milk, and coffee, which is high in carbohydrates and low in fat and protein. Blood sugar levels are monitored at several intervals to assess whether they drop significantly after the meal.

If professional testing is not an option, you can try a similar approach at home using a high-carb meal and a blood glucose monitor. Though not as precise as a medical test, this approach can reveal patterns, especially if symptoms consistently appear after eating high-carb foods.

2. Ambulatory Blood Glucose Monitoring

With a home glucose monitor, you can track blood sugar levels at different times of the day, especially when symptoms like shaking or dizziness appear. This self-monitoring method can be affordable and insightful. To do this, check your blood sugar level whenever you feel symptoms and record it in a food and symptom diary. By examining the timing of symptoms and glucose dips, you may identify specific foods or meals that trigger reactive hypoglycemia.

If a glucometer is beyond your budget, look for community resources or nonprofit organizations that provide free meters or strips for those managing blood sugar issues. Some pharmacies and manufacturers also offer discounts or assistance programs.

However, note that ambulatory testing has its limits: if symptoms occur while you're unable to check your levels, the data may be incomplete. Additionally, by the time you test, your body may already have begun compensating, leading to a normal or near-normal reading. Despite these drawbacks, self-testing remains one of the most accessible diagnostic tools for many people.

3. Oral Glucose Tolerance Test (OGTT)

The OGTT, primarily used to detect diabetes, may provide insights for diagnosing reactive hypoglycemia. This test involves fasting overnight, drinking a high-glucose liquid, and having blood drawn at intervals over a few hours to observe glucose changes.

OGTT is often costly without insurance and is generally not the best test for non-diabetic hypoglycemia. For those with insurance or access to low-cost clinics, discuss the option with your provider. Alternatively, you may find sliding-scale options or community health programs that offer OGTTs as part of diabetes screenings.

4. Fasting Plasma Glucose and A1C Testing

While fasting plasma glucose (FPG) and A1C tests are primarily used to diagnose diabetes, they can rule out or confirm glucose regulation issues. The FPG measures blood sugar levels after an overnight fast, while the A1C test provides an average blood sugar level over the last three months.

FPG and A1C tests are frequently available at low-cost health clinics or health fairs. For those struggling with the expense of full blood work, check for discounts or seek out community programs offering diabetes screenings that may include these tests.

5. The Whipple Triad

The Whipple Triad is a diagnostic approach used to confirm hypoglycemia by evaluating three key criteria:

- **Do you have physical symptoms** of hypoglycemia (like sweating or shaking)?

- **Does your blood glucose drop below a certain threshold** during these episodes?

- **Do symptoms resolve when blood glucose levels return to normal?**

Answering "yes" to all three questions strongly suggests

reactive hypoglycemia. This method is helpful for self-monitoring at home if medical tests are inaccessible, though it's always beneficial to confirm these findings with a healthcare professional when possible.

6. Vitamin and Mineral Screening

Nutritional deficiencies in vitamins and minerals, such as calcium, magnesium, and B vitamins, can contribute to hypoglycemic episodes. Ask your doctor to include these in your lab work if possible. For those without access to regular lab tests, consider investing in a quality multivitamin and adjusting your diet to include foods that help stabilize blood sugar, like leafy greens, lean proteins, and whole grains.

Many online labs offer affordable nutrient screening kits, and local health centers may provide free or reduced-cost screenings. Checking for deficiencies is an essential part of understanding your overall health and identifying potential triggers for blood sugar imbalances.

What happens if i dont get an official diagnosis and i try to treat it on its own?

If you try to manage reactive hypoglycemia on your own without an official diagnosis, there are a few potential risks and challenges. While lifestyle changes like balanced meals and regular blood sugar monitoring can help, they may not address underlying causes, leading to missed health issues or less effective symptom management. Here's what you might encounter:

1. Misidentifying the Cause

- Reactive hypoglycemia can stem from various conditions, such as prediabetes, insulin sensitivity, nutrient deficiencies, or, rarely, tumors like insulinoma. Without an official diagnosis, you might not pinpoint the true cause, leading to management strategies that address symptoms but miss the underlying problem.

- Some symptoms, like anxiety, weakness, and brain fog, can overlap with other conditions, such as anxiety disorders or thyroid issues, so there's a risk of confusing symptoms.

2. Missed Opportunity for a Tailored Treatment Plan

- A doctor can help create a plan specific to your needs, especially if tests reveal particular triggers, such as insulin spikes or low glucagon levels. Treating it on your own may lead to trial and error that delays effective relief.

- Certain conditions require specific treatments. For example, an underlying Helicobacter pylori infection can be treated with antibiotics, while deficiencies in magnesium or calcium might need supplementation.

3. Increased Risk of Long-term Health Issues

- For conditions like prediabetes, early intervention can prevent further progression to diabetes. Without knowing your diagnosis, you might miss early signs of developing metabolic issues, which can lead to long-term complications.

- If you have an insulinoma or another rare but treatable cause of hypoglycemia, treating symptoms alone could mean that the underlying condition worsens.

4. Potential Over-restriction of Diet

- Without clear guidance, you may over-restrict certain foods or essential nutrients. Some people might cut out carbohydrates too drastically, leading to low energy, mood changes, and other nutrient deficiencies.

- A doctor or dietitian can help balance your diet to control blood sugar without sacrificing essential nutrients.

5. Limited Symptom Relief

- Home strategies might help stabilize blood sugar temporarily but may not prevent all episodes. A diagnosis can provide insight into whether your blood sugar dips are due to insulin overproduction, poor liver glycogen stores, or food sensitivity, which may require different management strategies.

- Many people with reactive hypoglycemia feel immediate relief with small adjustments, but for lasting improvement, an official diagnosis can streamline your approach.

How to Start Treating Reactive Hypoglycemia on Your Own Safely

If a diagnosis isn't accessible, start by focusing on balanced, regular meals with protein, healthy fats, and complex carbohydrates. Track your symptoms and blood sugar levels to learn which foods help or trigger episodes. As you try these strategies, stay mindful of potential symptoms that could signal other health issues, and consult a healthcare provider if possible.

Conclusion: Establishing a Baseline with Step One

Getting a diagnosis is the foundation of your journey to manage reactive hypoglycemia. It's essential to establish a baseline so that you can effectively implement lifestyle changes that address the root cause of your symptoms. The tests and tools discussed here provide various paths to achieving clarity, whether through medical professionals or accessible, at-home methods.

In Step Two, we'll begin focusing on specific lifestyle strategies that stabilize blood sugar levels, manage symptoms, and support long-term health. By following this 5-Step Recovery Plan, you'll develop a structured approach to navigating and controlling reactive hypoglycemia day-to-day.

Step Two: Eliminate These Foods for Stable Blood Sugar

Adjusting your diet by eliminating specific foods can be transformative for managing reactive hypoglycemia, as well as improving overall health. Many people find that even small dietary changes lead to noticeable improvements, especially when processed and high-glycemic foods are replaced with nutrient-rich, whole foods. The following food list provides guidance on what to avoid to keep blood sugar stable.

Foods to Avoid

1. **Refined Grains and Processed Breads**

   - Products like white bread, bagels, pizza dough, burger buns, and other refined bread products can cause sharp blood sugar spikes followed by quick drops, which are particularly disruptive for those with hypoglycemia. During the refining process, these grains lose almost all fiber, which helps stabilize blood sugar.

- o **What to Choose Instead**: Substitute these with whole grain or sprouted grain breads. Whole grains digest more slowly, helping to prevent dramatic blood sugar swings.

2. **White Pasta**

   - o Traditional white pasta is made from refined flour, which is quickly broken down into sugar, potentially leading to blood sugar highs and lows.

   - o **What to Choose Instead**: Whole grain or legume-based pasta (such as chickpea or lentil pasta) are good alternatives. They provide more fiber and protein, helping to slow digestion and stabilize blood glucose.

3. **Sugary Breakfast Cereals**

   - o Most breakfast cereals contain added sugars, even those marketed as "healthy." These can create a rapid spike in blood sugar.

   - o **What to Choose Instead**: Opt for whole oats, bran, or unsweetened granola with added nuts and seeds. Adding a protein source, like nuts or Greek yogurt, further stabilizes blood sugar.

4. **Added Sugars and Syrups**

   - o Table sugar, maple syrup, honey, and high fructose corn syrup are all quick sources of glucose, causing a spike in blood sugar levels.

   - o **What to Choose Instead**: Use natural sweeteners like agave syrup sparingly and pair them with protein-rich foods to avoid quick blood sugar rises.

5. **Sweetened Plant Milks**

   - Some plant-based milks, like sweetened soy or rice milk, can contain added sugars.

   - **What to Choose Instead**: Unsweetened versions of almond, coconut, or oat milk are better options.

6. **Hidden Sugars in Packaged Foods**

   - Many packaged foods contain hidden sugars in ingredients like syrups, maltose, or fructose. Check labels on canned goods, yogurts, salad dressings, sauces, and soups to see if they contain added sugars.

   - **What to Choose Instead**: Look for "unsweetened" or "no added sugar" options. Making some of these items, like salad dressings and sauces, from scratch is an excellent way to avoid hidden sugars.

7. **Sodas and Sugary Drinks**

   - Sodas, fruit juices, and even diet sodas can lead to blood sugar instability. Research suggests that artificial sweeteners can disrupt insulin regulation.

   - **What to Choose Instead**: Water, herbal teas, or sparkling water with a splash of lemon or a hint of natural fruit flavor provide hydrating, sugar-free alternatives.

8. **Pastries, Cakes, and Sweets**

- These treats contain high amounts of refined sugar and carbohydrates, causing a quick rise and subsequent crash in blood sugar.

- **What to Choose Instead**: If you crave something sweet, try a small portion of dark chocolate (70% cacao or higher) or a homemade dessert made with alternative sweeteners and whole ingredients.

9. **Restaurant Foods and Takeout**

- Many restaurant dishes contain hidden sugars, especially in sauces, dressings, and glazes.

- **What to Choose Instead**: If dining out, opt for grilled proteins and request any sauces on the side. Whole foods like steamed vegetables or plain grains are usually better choices than entrees with sauces or dressings.

10. **White Potatoes and High-Glycemic Starches**

- Foods like baked potatoes, fries, and potato chips can cause blood sugar spikes.

- **What to Choose Instead**: Sweet potatoes, with their higher fiber content, or other low-glycemic vegetables like cauliflower are good substitutes. Small amounts of potatoes in soups or stews, where they're paired with proteins, are fine in moderation.

11. **High-Sugar Fruits**

- While fruits contain natural sugars, they can still spike blood glucose levels, especially when eaten in large quantities.

- o **What to Choose Instead**: Pair small portions of low-glycemic fruits, like berries, with a protein like yogurt or nuts to slow down sugar absorption.

12. **Coffee and Alcohol**

- o Both coffee and alcohol can interfere with blood sugar stability, especially on an empty stomach.

- o **What to Choose Instead**: If you enjoy these beverages, try having them alongside a balanced meal with protein and fat to buffer the impact on blood sugar. Herbal teas or chicory coffee alternatives offer non-stimulant options that are easier on blood sugar.

What to Do in a Blood Sugar Emergency

In cases of a blood sugar drop, it's essential to choose foods that will provide fast relief without triggering another low. If you have diabetes or experience severe hypoglycemia symptoms, take immediate action to raise blood sugar, such as:

- **For Immediate Sugar Needs**:
  - o Glucose tablets or gels (follow instructions on packaging)
  - o 4 ounces of juice or soda (non-diet)
  - o 1 tablespoon of sugar, honey, or corn syrup

- **If You're Not Diabetic**: Consuming pure sugar may cause a rebound effect, leading to another crash. Instead, pair a carbohydrate with a protein to stabilize blood sugar. Here are a few combinations to consider:

- o **Milk and Cheese**: Milk provides quick sugars, while cheese offers fat and protein to keep blood sugar stable.

- o **Yogurt with Nuts**: Plain yogurt with nuts slows the release of sugar into the bloodstream.

- o **Nut Butter on Whole Grain Toast**: Whole grain toast with almond or peanut butter combines fiber and protein for sustained energy.

- o **A Small Cup of Juice with Fish or Eggs**: The juice gives you a quick sugar boost, while the protein in fish or eggs helps prevent a sudden crash.

Benefiting from These Choices

By eliminating refined carbohydrates, sugary foods, and processed products, you're not only managing reactive hypoglycemia but also improving your body's overall function. **Everyone can benefit from these food choices**, as they help stabilize energy levels, improve mental clarity, and support long-term metabolic health. Whether you're dealing with reactive hypoglycemia, insulin sensitivity, or just seeking a balanced diet, focusing on fresh, unprocessed foods is key to lasting health.

What's Next?

Now that you understand which foods to avoid and how to manage emergencies, the next step in your recovery journey involves learning how to build a blood sugar-friendly diet that works for you. In the upcoming chapters, you'll dive into practical meal planning strategies, balanced food choices, and how to create a sustainable eating routine that keeps your energy steady all day.

Discover more in *Reactive Hypoglycemia: Your 5-Step Recovery Plan* by Allison Francis, MAT & Betty Johnson, MD (Ed.) Available now on Amazon and other major book retailers.